The Experiential Therapist

The Experiential Therapist

Phenomenology, Trauma-Informed Care, and Mental Health

Peter D. Ladd

LEXINGTON BOOKS
Lanham • Boulder • New York • London

Published by Lexington Books
An imprint of The Rowman & Littlefield Publishing Group, Inc.
4501 Forbes Boulevard, Suite 200, Lanham, Maryland 20706
www.rowman.com

6 Tinworth Street, London SE11 5AL, United Kingdom

British Library Cataloguing in Publication Information Available

Library of Congress Cataloging-in-Publication Data Available

Library of Congress Control Number: 2020942617
ISBN 978-1-7936-1901-3 (cloth)
ISBN 978-1-7936-1902-0 (electronic)

Dedicated to
Kinzlee Williams, Kyle Blanchfield and Dorian Ladd

Contents

Preface

Over the past number years in establishing and running mental health clinics, two issues jump out at me. First, the thinking found in medical practice, and the psychiatrists who advocate for it have dominated the field of mental health. Second, the rest of us, psychologists, mental health counselors, clinical social workers, trauma therapists, and so on, have to figure out how our training fits into this medically oriented practice. The present reality is that many professionals other than psychiatrists simply adjust to a more psychiatric model, while we go back and forth between what is required by a medical model and at the same time try to fit in thinking that does not solely rely on medical practice.

Also, as someone who has trained graduate-level mental health counselors for many years, my desire has been to fit a holistic, alternative way of thinking into a more medical model form of practice before students graduate. Even though thinking from a medical perspective has moved forward the field of mental health and has gained respectable success, it seems shortsighted to hold on to a "one-size-fits-all" approach. Limiting ourselves as professionals to one perspective points more to standardization rather than diversity regarding our human condition. In the following chapters a different way of looking at and thinking about client/patients in mental health will be the major theme. Here is a basic preface leading to this goal.

The most common thinking in the field of medicine and specifically mental health are as follows: What is most important regarding mental health practice for the therapist is the diagnostic symptoms that make up a mental disorder. Symptoms are connected to how one thinks, what one feels, and how one behaves. Treatment means managing a cluster of symptoms while trying to minimize the damage and, in so doing, making life tolerable and patients tolerable to other people. The use of the Diagnostic and Statistical

Manual (DSM), especially the latest version the DSM 5 (2013), continues to move mental suffering closer to the field of medicine. In a very real sense, a patient is considered being outside of normal, much as the thinking behind high blood pressure being abnormal.

What symptoms a patient possesses means accepting a disorder and learning to live with it. Succinctly put, patients live within a symptoms reduction, symptoms maintenance model. Reducing symptoms through a diagnostic-oriented treatment is the ultimate goal, and with disorders that have a clear biological base, such as schizophrenia, bipolar disorder, autism, and others, the strict medical model has proven moderately successful. Where it becomes confusing are those disorders such as anxiety, or mood disorders, and others that may be symptomatic of deeper underlying traumas that have affected the brain, and the human experiences connected to them (Pai, Suris, and North 2018).

There is an alternative way of thinking, and it keeps growing as patients in mental health become better-informed and continue to find meaning in their personal experiences. In response to this new awareness, experiential thinkers make a 180-degree turn toward a client's experience of mental suffering. What becomes important is the meaning found in stressful and traumatic life experiences, not symptoms related to any mental disorder. During the pain and suffering in one's everyday world, disruptive levels of stress and trauma can happen. In therapy, this may lead to a more holistic perspective that affects a client experientially (Ho, Ngai, Wu, and Hou 2018).

Experiential thought is about setting the stage for future experiences, not a systematic diagnosis and treatment of a present disorder. It warns against life experiences becoming pathologies. It advocates that working through stress and trauma will create hope, resilience, and self-esteem. People, places, and things may leave clients scarred, but what is done in collaboration with a more experiential therapist helps create new possibilities. Clients have the ability to learn from their scars whether it is happening in the outside world or within one's brain, and with the wisdom learned in both of these areas, clients can improve their lives.

Unfortunately, as I said previously, most of the mental health system in the United States is dominated by thinking based on medicine and is controlled by a psychiatric perspective (Elkins 2007). In this respect, experiential thinking has a distinct cultural disadvantage. It follows a different path not necessarily accepted by both mainstream therapists and patients. This is relevant when patients become more concerned with their diagnosis than following their personal experiences. In the defense of patients, medically oriented thoughts can become bigger than the people using them. Sometimes to receive help, patients need insurance reimbursements and diagnostic labels to carry on their everyday lives. This may cloud their experiences and accept a pathology based on economic and bureaucratic reasons.

Because of this, a patient may fall into the trap of accepting a diagnostic label cloaked in a blanket of medicine, and eventually working that label into their identity—making pathology a major role in their own thinking. Such patients may become the "frequent flyers" of the mental health industry, spending multiple visits to institutions serving their pathological views of themselves. On the other hand, using experiential thought in the practice of mental health may require awareness and courage from both the client and the therapist. Unfortunately, medical model thinking in present-day cultural norms advocate for compliance rather than courage. The reality is that experiential thinking by clients and therapists faces not only opposition by medical model practitioners but also cultural pressure to remain in the realm of medicine. This is principally based on the popular mythology that psychiatric thinking is the ultimate and only answer, rather than pursuing thoughts that emphasize client meaningful experiences. When you think about it, clients using experiential thinking have to consider the courage that may be required to work through the pain and suffering of what is happening in traumatic life experiences, while many times being offered the "quick fix" of psychotropic drugs. This may be a tall order for patients who historically have relied on practices controlled by experts who encourage patients to be compliant.

This raises the issue of whether it is possible to grow and change when using experiential thought. One of the most powerful mental health practices in favor of an experiential alternative is the priority given to the therapeutic relationship, and research continuously backs its importance (Jacobsen 2016). Simply put, client growth and change may not happen without it. In spite of these difficulties, more experiential thought seems to be the alternative advocated by mental health professionals who believe in personal identity, choice, empowerment, and when the unique experiences of their clients are more important than recognizing a standardized disorder. For example, in the field of trauma therapy, a diagnosis is less important than how clients eventually face overwhelming moments that changed their brains and bodies, and eventually changed their lives.

One of the questions that the following chapters brings to the forefront, "Can disorders based on empirical thinking found in the medical model make room for experiential thinking, and can an alternative way of thinking help to improve the present state of mental health?"

Before answering that question, the following pages make comparisons between thinking that focuses on finding meaning in people's life experiences and thinking where relieving symptoms is the ultimate goal. With this in mind, one repeated theme in each chapter will be the description of the medical model system itself, which contains fact-finding, diagnosis, treatment through drugs, therapeutic techniques, treatment planning, and medical model therapy. My hope is that the redundancy of themes does not distract you from the message being conveyed in each chapter. The medical model system itself forces professionals in the field of mental health into a certain manner of thinking promoted by the procedures found in natural science. So, each chapter is not to decide which way of thinking is more effective but gain a perspective on an alternative way of thinking that may be relevant for a more human science, a science that values human experience. In sorting through all of this, it is the hope that something can be learned regarding our present mental health system and how professionals seek answers and choices for client/patient suffering.

On a personal note, such experiential thinking may be particularly relevant with the emblematic experience of COVID-19. Where beyond the physical crisis lies the mental one for all of us caught in such an experience. Where receiving a mental health diagnosis and label falls short of each person's individual experience. Where *working through traumatic experiences* may be more relevant than *being diagnosed with mental disorders*. Where *sharing these experiences* may be the first step to recovery. Where during this time of uncertainty cultural change may include the mental health profession.

Peter D. Ladd
St. Lawrence University
August 31, 2020

Acknowledgments

I would like to thank those clients from different mental health clinics who inspired the case studies in this book. I changed specific names and locations in each case study to protect the anonymity of those willing to help. However, it also is important to note that practicing phenomenology or trauma-informed care was evident with those therapists and counselors who understood the importance of human dialogue and experience.

I would like to thank these institutions for their belief in another method of practicing talk therapy and how it can improve the practice of mental health beyond a medical model. In this regard, I want to acknowledge Linda Zerbe, vice president of Student Affairs at Desales University, for her holistic approach to the administration of Student Affairs. Her understanding at the university level could act as a model for universities looking for a more experiential approach.

Acknowledgments go out to Tish Jepsen, Penn State University, Berks, for her tireless effort and commitment to students and their futures. Her understanding of the whole person experience is responsible for student success when leaving the university by looking at the world from a more experiential perspective.

Kyle E. Blanchfield, JD, took the time to edit this book and has helped in other projects as an editor and coauthor. She demonstrates leadership from an experiential point of view, leading to higher levels of critical thinking for leadership students. I would also like to thank her tireless effort in promoting diversity and social justice from a fair experiential perspective.

Special thanks go out to my friend and colleague Mike Elberty, a phenomenologist extraordinaire who comes from a family of critical thinkers. Especially, his father Bill Elberty who guided me in my youth as a mentor and colleague. The dialogue between us continues now that I find myself in the role that his father played in my personal development. Such history deserves recognition, and both Bill and Mike need to be recognized for some of the ideas found in this manuscript.

I must mention Don Moncrief from Duquesne University who took the time in directing a curious Vietnam War veteran many years ago into the field of psychology. His inspiration was at the beginning of a long career where I am still experiencing the influence of his words. As a Jesuit priest who spent twelve years in silence before taking up the professoriate, I commend his discipline and courage.

Acknowledgments go out to River Hospital, Canton-Potsdam Hospital, the Counseling Centers of Northern New York, Clarkson University Counseling Center, St. Lawrence University Counseling Center, the SUNY Canton Counseling Center, Hospice of St. Lawrence County, the St. Lawrence Psychiatric Center, and the Holistic Health and Wellness Program for their practice and belief in therapy beyond a medical model.

James T. Hansen, Oakland University, needs to be given a big thank-you for his support. Structurally, I have not met anyone finer in describing the culture of the phenomenological/humanistic movement. He also helped solidify my thoughts in more human terms and directed me away from more esoteric explanations.

I would also like to mention AnnMarie Churchill, who was my colleague for many years where her friendship was as important to me as the wisdom she shared on a continuous basis. The work she is doing with the COVID-19 pandemic in Canada should be recognized, so I am taking this opportunity to do just that. When I think about experiential therapists her name is the first to come to mind. Our work together with Native people is still one of the highlights of my career.

Finally, to my mentors Viktor Frankl and Carl Rogers who turned out to be two of the most down-to-earth people that I have experienced. They were all about the dialogue whether academically or just sitting around at the end of the day and enjoying each other's company. I am still amazed how certain people make up one's identity just by the good fortune of having an opportunity to experience them. Though these great leaders are gone, some of us still help their influence live on by a commitment to the human experience, and all of its mysteries.

Chapter 1

Mental Health Thinking

What is the definition of mental health thinking? Defining such thinking brings one back to Sigmund Freud, at the start of his first of *Five Lectures* at Clark University in 1909, where Freud celebrates the presence of so many nonmedical people in the audience (Freud and Starchy 1989). He goes on to differentiate his new method of psychoanalysis—the talking cure—from medicine and begins a long history where patient experience through talk therapy becomes a driving force in the field of mental health. Freud's form of psychoanalysis was designed to release pent-up or repressed emotions and memories or to lead the client to catharsis, or healing (McLeod 2014). This goal was for Freud, and still is, accomplished through talking to another person about the big questions in life, the things that matter, and diving into the complexities of human experience, and especially traumatic experiences that lie beneath the conscious mind.

Even though Freud eventually developed theories around the unconscious mind, it was the experiences of patients that promoted these theories. Others such as Alfred Adler and his Individual Psychology, a more holistic/humanistic approach, or Carl Jung's focusing on the collective unconscious, a more spiritual approach, along with Freud became the baseline for talk therapy through the first half of the twentieth century. Their differences in theories did not deter from their willingness to talk with patients about their experiences. Beyond any medical model procedures for mental health recovery was the "Talk Therapy" models. Later in the twentieth century such figures as Carl Rogers, focusing on a more humanistic form of talk therapy, or Rollo May, focusing more on an existential/phenomenological form of talk therapy, continued to treat client/patients' experiences from their individual perspectives, recognizing the importance of experience in discovering each new theory and each new theoretical practice.

There are hundreds of psychotherapy approaches or schools of thought. By 1980 there were more than 250, by 1996 more than 450, and at the start of the twenty-first century there were over a 1,000 different named psychotherapies—some being minor variations while others are based on very different conceptions of psychology, ethics (how to live), or technique. All of which begin with the experience of the client in some way whether it is behavioral, cognitive, neurological, social, or emotional. In practice, therapy is often not of one pure type but draws from a number of perspectives and schools. Furthermore, the importance of the therapeutic relationship, also known as therapeutic alliance, between client and therapist is often regarded as crucial to psychotherapy. Obviously, one could go on and on about others practicing and developing their personal brand of psychotherapy, especially about human experience and its impact in the field of mental health. These brief examples exemplify many other thoughtful practitioners who developed their theories around the experiences of human beings and added to the literature of talk therapy and its indelible impact on mental health. (For the purposes of this book, phenomenological and trauma-informed care forms of psychotherapy are chosen from *my* personal experiences.)

However, in the 1950s a movement that was instigated by psychiatrists with the introduction of the antidepressant Prozac resulted in the ultimate decline in the popularity of talk therapy models. Psychotropic medicine now made psychiatrists "true" medical doctors where they could treat patients like any other doctor in the field of medicine, and eventually psychotropic medication was complimented by the institutionalization of empirically validated treatment (EVT) that has led to evidence-based practices. In 1992 Division 29 (Psychotherapy) under David Barlow endorsed the proposal that all treatments should target DSM symptoms and be compared with medications in controlled clinical trials. In 1995 the American Psychological Association endorsed this vision. They started to create a list of "approved treatments" for specific diagnoses and symptoms, and it was argued that all psychologists should be retrained to "administer" EVTs according to carefully written manuals. The argument, derived from the pharmaceutical model of research, was that treatments should be administered precisely and objectively. Any reference to the personal qualities of the therapist or experiential information from the patients was treated as a statistically "confounding variable" (Duncan 2012).

The age of the medical model in the treatment of mental disorders had begun. Talk therapy and more specifically client/patient experiences were marginalized by a mental health industry that was controlled by medical model thinking, insurance companies, and Big Pharma. The thinking behind mental health professionals had turned toward the practice of medicine. Yet, to be fair, there was significant opposition from Division 32 (Humanistic

Psychology) and Division 39 (Psychoanalysis) and numerous excellent publications in relevant journals. Research also started to come in which increasingly undermined the assumptions underlying the medical model approach to talk therapy—largely reduced to cognitive behavioral therapy (CBT) (Adams 2020). Bruce Wampold's book, *The Great Psychotherapy Debate*, came out in 2000 and it marked a turn back to talk therapy and experiential thinking (Wampold 2000).

In 2005 American Psychiatric Association's (APA) task force on psychotherapy under the leadership of Ron Levant reinstated the therapeutic relationship as essential to the process of psychotherapy, and in doing so, reinstated the therapist's expertise and authority in clinical decision-making. It also reinstated that dialogue and collaboration are foundational in any therapeutic relationship—not prescribed symptom removal. Despite this, much of the culture of psychological treatment has soldiered on within the rhetoric and logic of the medical model: practitioners as diagnosticians and the applicants of symptom-focused treatments (Adams 2020).

Taking all of this into consideration, where exactly do we stand in present-day mental health and what is the definition of mental health thinking in present-day mental health practice? From this brief history of talk therapy, it becomes obvious that there are possibly hundreds of perspectives regarding mental health thinking according to the history of talk therapy regarding human experience. Therefore, I would like to give my definition of mental health thinking from an experiential perspective. Having had the honor and privilege of developing two different mental health clinics and having worked in both, one a medical model, the other a more experiential model, I want to share my experience from both perspectives and why I believe mental health thinking should return to equal prominence between experiential thinking and medical model thinking. I believe the time has come for equality in the field of mental health. Beyond the different theories and beyond those talk therapy practitioners of these theories lies one connecting thread, namely client/patient experiences. The following four models demonstrate both an experiential and medical model perspective in the field of mental health.

MEDICAL MODEL THINKING

Classic Medical Model Thinking

Classic medical model thinking is a biological approach to psychopathology where disorders have an organic or physical cause. The focus of this thinking is on genetics, neurotransmitters, neurophysiology, neuroanatomy, and so on (Deacon 2013). The approach argues that mental disorders are related to the physical structure and functioning of the brain. Behaviors such as delusions are symptoms of mental illness, as is suicidal ideation, or extreme fears, such as phobias about spiders and so on. Different illnesses can be identified as clusters of symptoms that go together and are caused by the illness in areas of the body. These symptoms lead the psychiatrist in making a diagnosis, for example, this patient is suffering from a severe psychosis. He is suffering from the medical condition we call schizophrenia.

The thinking that takes place in a classic medical model is by an expert, usually in mental health a psychiatrist who makes a judgment of the patient's behavior, through a clinical interview after some form of referral is made. The expert will judge that the patient is exhibiting abnormal behavior by asking questions and by patient observation. This model includes history, mental examination, ancillary assessment if needed, diagnosis, treatment, and prognosis with or without treatment (Nesse and Stein 2012). In the realm of physical ailments, it is difficult to name an alternative to medical diagnosis and treatment. However, does this model hold true for psychological ailments as well?

Classic medical model thinking is characterized by a reductionist approach that attributes mental illness to a single cause located within the body (Wade and Halligan 2017). In classic medical model thinking in mental health, it is most likely located in the brain or nervous system. This is the model that most people refer to when they say "medical model" from a layperson's perspective. In the field of psychiatry, this model has been proven effective, especially in treating schizophrenia, bipolar disorder, and other more biologically based mental illnesses.

There are many schools of thought about the medical model in the psychiatry world. Supporters of this type of thinking usually consider symptoms to be signs of the inner physical disorder, usually in the brain, and believe that if symptoms are connected, they can be characterized by a diagnostic label. The biological approach of the medical model focuses on genetics, neurotransmitters, neurophysiology, neuroanatomy, and so on (Deacon 2013). Psychopathology says that disorders have an organic or physical cause. The approach suggests that mental conditions are related to the brain's physical structure and functioning.

Symptoms of mental illness, such as bipolar disorder, are given a label caused by these symptoms. These labels allow a psychiatrist to make a diagnosis and prescribe treatment. Based on the medical model, mental illness should be treated, in part, as a medical condition, typically through the use of prescription medications. It must be noted that medications for mental illness change brain chemistry. In most cases, these medications add or modify a chemical that is responsible for problems with mood, perception, anxiety, or other issues. In the correct dosage, medication can have an acceptable impact on functioning.

However, its greatest everyday usage is in the treatment of common mood and anxiety disorders not diagnosed by psychiatrists but by general practitioners in the field of medicine. Despite the fact that one in four visits to primary care are for psychiatric-related complaints, these providers typically have little specific training in psychiatry and follow a way of thinking that may not be related to a psychiatric medical model (Fluery 2012). After medical school and residency, much of their psychiatric education is delivered by pharmaceutical representatives (Whittchen 2003). There are no specific procedures connected to the classic medical model thinking in mental health. It is more in the realm of marketing. Pharmaceutical companies try to inform general practitioners of how psychotropic drugs can help other areas of care based on the marketplace for these drugs.

Obtaining a prescription for psychotropic drugs before a formal mental health evaluation has been performed can be quite risky. Also, in psychiatry, there are many symptoms that overlap with other disorders, so the same symptom can represent more than one disorder, making diagnosis a tentative enterprise of experimentation with possible numerous drugs until the correct drug is found effective. Additionally, if there are multiple diagnoses occurring together, a fairly common scenario, sometimes a medication helps one condition but makes another one worse.

It is interesting to note that commercials regarding psychotropic drugs in the media will refer to the side effects of these drugs but do little to inform the thinking of consumers that research shows that most of them work in conjunction with mental health therapy (Baroud 2016). As previously stated, the classic medical model seems to be used, at least some of it, by general practitioners in the field of medicine. Having said that, in severe cases of psychosis and other chronic situations, psychotropic drugs have helped a majority of patients given these labels. Neuroscience and the pharmaceutical companies through their research have supplied the classic medical model thinking with a blueprint for gathering information, making a diagnosis, developing a treatment, and following on treatment to reduce symptoms of these disorders.

Bio/Psycho/Social Medical Model Thinking

Over the years there have been classical medical model therapists who have questioned strict medical model thinking. These were experts that did not choose to abandon it but wanted to make it more humanistic. Their thinking led to what is now known as a bio/psycho/social medical model. These practitioners take into account the social context in which patients live, how they feel, think, believe, and behave. This does not do away with the "bio" part of medicine, but it does incorporate an entire domain of human existence that had been neglected, like interpersonal relationships, intergenerational trauma, adverse childhood experiences, stress, and so on (Engel 1997).

If you believe that mental health deserves to be researched and treated according to the best available empirical evidence, but you do not like dehumanizing or oppressing people, the bio/psycho/social approach to diagnosis should be appealing. In this way of thinking, clinicians use the DSM as one of several assessment tools within the context of interpersonal therapeutic conversations. Diagnosing someone as depressed does not necessarily mean the client is not given a pathology. As long as the client is treated with empathy, unconditional positive regard, and genuineness as a unique human being, having a psychiatric label is acceptable.

In 1977, the American pathologist and psychiatrist George Engel published in the *Journal of Science* his paper "The Need for a New Medical Model: A Challenge for Biomedicine," introducing the term "bio/psycho/social model" (Smith 2012). This model based on the results of Engel's studies in depression and psychogenic pain, constituted a challenge for biomedicine and the biomedical model. The basic principles of the model included the biological, psychological, and social dimensions of the person's life, and the perception that the person suffers as a whole and not through isolated organs. The doctor should use a holistic approach regarding illness and should consider his/her relations with the patient as socially equal. The personality and the emotions of the patient, as well as the particular environmental conditions in which the person lives in, should be taken into account.

There is no doubt that the bio/psycho/social model has established a more empathetic and compassionate approach in medical practice (Engel 1997). Hans Selye emphasized in his research that psychological stressful factors may have injurious consequences on health, while the response systems to stress may deregulate not only by genetic factors but also from experiences and stressful life events (Selye 1976). This gives credence to considering human experience. Psychosocial factors may co-determine the patient's vulnerability and the illness's severity.

The bio/psycho/social thinker considers the interactions with genetic susceptibility, personality, stressful events, and, generally, with the patient's social context. Yet, environmental factors do not change the probability of being labeled with a mental disorder. The rules are strict regarding this model. Nonadherence to pharmacology, as well as to psychosocial interventions, may cause a defective recovery and recurrence of the disorder, as well as insufficient use of mental health resources. Though a more humanistic approach is suggested in this model, the thinking from many of its practitioners still hold on to perceiving themselves as experts, and their thoughts are intended to work from a predetermined treatment plan.

From more classical thinking psychiatrists, the bio/psycho/social model has been criticized that it does not constitute a scientific or philosophical model; it does not provide an answer to the crucial question of how the biological, psychological, and social variables interact in the expression of a disease; it does not provide guidance on the exact time of its application; and finally, it allows for a wide range of interventions without providing specific guidelines of concrete therapeutic treatment plans (Benning 2015).

Regarding the way one thinks about patients in this model is based on beliefs that a more humanistic approach is important but still going back to a more classic medical model way of thinking when developing a treatment plan. For these reasons, the bio/psycho/social way of thinking is particularly applicable in psychiatric disorders but only recognizes more humanistic practices as secondary concerns. The bio/psycho/social model, despite the criticism, continues to offer valuable clinical, educational, and research services, as well as to provide an important contribution to the formation of health policies, not only for psychiatry but for the whole of medicine as well (Kusnanto et al. 2018).

The one spin-off of the bio/psycho/social model is the recovery model where the clinician is envisioned more as a collaborator rather than an authority. An important critique of the bio/psycho/social approach from a recovery perspective is that it still positions the clinician as being best-equipped, rather than the client to appraise a clinical scenario by applying theoretical and technical knowledge. The therapist's version, while aiming to be collaborative, may be privileged above that of the client (MacDonald and Mikes-Liu 2012).

EXPERIENTIAL MODEL THINKING

Phenomenological Thinking

(Note: The following phenomenological thinking is influenced by my personal experiences over the years and does not necessarily adhere to classic phenomenological theory. It may be that your style of phenomenological thinking differs from my approach. Feel free to differ or revise this approach according to your personal experiences in mental health. It seems contradictory to me in not allowing one's personal experiences to be a part of a phenomenological perspective.)

Phenomenological model of mental health is firmly based on human experience. It proceeds through careful description and aims to explore people's difficulties in the experience of living rather than by referring to psycho-diagnostic categories, or other theoretical concepts. It seeks to achieve understanding by encouraging a person to set his or her problems against the wider horizon of the human condition. It avoids prescription, interpretation, explanation and emphasizes description of purpose, meaning, values, conflicts, dilemmas, and paradoxes instead (Deurzen 2015).

In many respects, phenomenological thinking in mental health is a reaction and a defense against the empirical and measurable nature found in the medical model. It takes a position based on a more experiential perspective where it becomes impossible to evaluate patients' mental problems only on what is objective and measurable. It contends that much of human experience is based on unmeasurable nuances unique to each individual along with their unique life experiences, and it may be these unique nuances that make the difference in recovery. A client who comes to a phenomenologically oriented therapist can expect the focus initially will remain on the client. He or she has the opportunity to tell their story and those experiences that brought them to therapy in the first place. The client and therapist continue by focusing on what dialogue develops spontaneously. There is no pre-diagnosis or treatment plan. During the course of therapy these activities will emerge on their own. The more the phenomenologically oriented therapist attunes to the client, she or he begins developing higher possibility in forming therapeutic alliance. That alliance is the key to this model of therapy. Without it the dialogue between client and therapist can turn into a fact-finding experience, where the flow of the conversation is replaced with a more structured form of communication, usually initiated by a more expert-driven discussion. It becomes important in this way of thinking for the dialogue to speak on its own terms. The famous philosopher Martin Buber might describe dialogue as having three elements: the client, the therapist, and the dialogue itself. There are a number of well-established theories that sound similar to this thinking (Buber 2007). Carl Roger's person-centered therapy allows the dialogue to flow, however, with more of a focus on the client's words than the dialogue between client and therapist (Rogers 2003).

Nevertheless, this model and others such as humanistic psychotherapy and contemporary psychoanalysis have in common the importance of the therapeutic alliance and the belief that a diagnosis should not be predetermined but should emerge from the interchange between client and therapist. In this manner, what is talked about or what techniques are used resonate in the meaning the clients and therapist attach to these activities. Another point to make is the assertion that phenomenological thinking emphasizes the subjective reality of individual existence, individual freedom, individual choice, and an emphasis on each person finding their own way in life by making personal choices and decisions.

Motivation for change does not necessarily come from compliance to the wishes of a therapist or a psychiatrist. Motivation for change comes from client awareness in meaningful ways. When the client combines learned knowledge with experiential wisdom and accepts the unique connection of experiential patterns in everyday living, a new accuracy and a new perspective becomes a possibility for the client. If a phenomenologically oriented therapist uses human experience to help the client grow and change, then it becomes meaningful for the client (Ladd 2018).

The Trauma-Informed Care Model of Thinking

(Note: The following trauma-informed care thinking is based on my personal experiences over the years and reflects my approach to trauma-informed care. This is how I see it. Feel free to allow your experiences to view it differently. However, the common ground is held in one's ability to work through trauma rather than believing it is a mental disorder.)

Another model that may be understood as an experiential actually deals with suffering and trauma from a more personal perspective, thus bases much of its thinking toward life experiences. The trauma model for therapy makes the assumption that instead of focusing on a diagnosis and a cluster of symptoms, it is more important to focus on a client's traumatic experiences. It is not what is wrong with you but what has happened to you. Focusing instantly on these experiences may lead to further trauma, and this is where experiential thinking can be valuable. To avoid this happening, the trauma therapist spends a significant amount of time creating safety for the client (Banitt 2019). In a sense, this mirrors the importance of the therapeutic alliance in phenomenological and humanistic thinking. Some of the themes that frequently emerge are the trouble surrounding attachment or the lack of it, when children do not form strong attachments with adults during early experiences, or disassociation when someone is traumatized to the extent that she or he forms emotional buffers to the outside world (Banitt 2019). In both of these traumas, the client should be treated cautiously until feeling safe. It is one thing to diagnose for attachment and disassociation disorders. It is quite another for a client to find meaning in working through these experiences.

A major issue to consider in a trauma model way of thinking is the damage of stressful life experiences that impact the body itself. These experiences have disruptive consequences playing out in neurological and sensory networks, the nervous system that connects many parts of the body including the brain and the gut (van der Kolk 2015). Much like the connection between everyday experience and phenomenology, a trauma model also combines empirical and experiential thinking that gets to the root of life experiences.

Again, early work should focus on restoring a sense of safety, but also for somatic reasons. Forming this bond, whether it is through safety or a therapeutic alliance, neurologically leads to self-regulation. Human memory is a sensory experience (van der Kolk 2015). Through longtime research, and innovation in trauma treatment, van der Kolk shares what he is learning about how the body works through trauma. He states the following:

> I think trauma really does confront you with the best and the worst. You see the horrendous things that people do to each other, but you also see resiliency, the power of love, the power of caring, the power of commitment, the power of commitment to oneself, the knowledge that there are things that are larger than our individual survival. And in some ways, I don't think you can appreciate the glory of life unless you also know the dark side of life. (van der Kolk 2015)

This statement alone emphasizes the same commitment as an experiential thinker. While medical model thinking wants to get rid of all suffering, experiential thinking separates necessary from unnecessary suffering, and so does trauma-informed care, in a trauma model of therapy.

There are other reasons that trauma therapy can be tied to experiential thinking. The use of mindfulness in trauma work is one example. Though many see mindfulness as a method, however it is more than that. It can be a way of thinking about everyday life. Mindfulness is paying attention, on purpose, to our moment-to-moment unfolding experiences in the present in a nonjudgmental manner. It is becoming aware of emerging experiences. This facilitates a receptive stance toward our emerging thoughts, feelings, emotions, body sensations, and noticing what is present in our world (Nanda 2009). It also works well with clients going through trauma. This makes most of it a more authentic experience.

Eye Movement Desensitization and Reprocessing (EMDR) is a neurological/experiential method (Riddle 2012). Though favoring neuroscience, it also is experiential by letting certain "dug-in" neural pathways be disrupted and normalized without any preconceived notions or plans. These examples and others fit more closely with a more experiential thought process than medical model thinking, especially when they are used in conjunction with an ongoing dialogue between client and therapist.

DISCUSSION

It is stated or referred to in all the above models that in mental health culture experiential thinking has a place and a purpose. Maybe not to the extent that it threatens the mainstream medical model culture but as a serious addition to it. We are in an age where talking directly to each other is becoming more difficult. Though social media has introduced many new ways of communicating, it has taken its toll on face-to-face dialogue and the healing that can accompany it. Such communication patterns are being tested by the recent COVID-19 crisis. This may require reasons for pointing out personal experiences of suffering in a more innovative and experiential manner. Such experiences are pointed out in the rest of this book. You will *not* learn an introductory course in either phenomenology or trauma-informed care but experiences of using them in the practice of the experiential therapist.

The Black Plague that threatened the inhabitants of this planet during medieval times was amazingly followed by the Renaissance. We may be in a similar position as we try to figure out a world in transition. My belief is that it may be an opportunity for some creative changes in the field of mental health. Or, maybe the current experiences will make those changes for us. Hopefully, some of this book may help in making the possibility for change a more realistic endeavor. Especially, for those client/patients who want their life-changing experiences to mean something.

Chapter 2

A Comparison

Let us look at two different methods of practicing mental health therapy. The first works from an empirical method, most notably practiced in a medical model where talking to patients is a part of a package that includes a collection of patient history, psychiatric diagnosis, possible pharmaceutical prescriptions, and a treatment plan that may include talk therapy and therapy techniques. It is a model that is expert-driven, based on a reductionistic formula that seeks to locate a cluster of symptoms that labels patients through the use of the Diagnostic and Statistical Manual 5 (DSM5) (Barsky 2017). In this manner, therapy takes on a peculiar form of presupposed discussion based on fact-finding that is not prepared for constant free-flowing dialogue.

During actual practice, in the collection of a patient's history no real dialogue is intended. It is a structured procedure to gather information for an upcoming psychiatric diagnosis, which also is a gathering of information made by experts with similar limitations on dialogue. The talking that takes place is expert-driven leading eventually to a psychological treatment plan. Talk therapy may enter the scene at this point but not necessarily to include dialogue from a patient's point of view. The talking to patients or patients talking to therapists, post-treatment plan is an expert-driven form of talking and may be effective to a certain degree if the presumed treatment plan is accurate—but even at that point, may be meaningful for the therapist and not necessarily for the patient. What happens when it is not accurate or when it helps reduce symptoms but has little effect on someone's personal life experiences?

The aforementioned description of the medical model regarding therapy does not fit all cases and all circumstances. There are highly qualified medical model therapists who take every opportunity to include the patient in the mental health process, and therefore practice a form of experiential thinking. However, structurally from the threshold of a scientific practice, the medical model's interest and direction for therapy is formulated around the diagnosis and treatment plan (Barsky 2017). So, no matter what the patient talks about or attempts to convey in their narrative during therapy, the therapist must keep in mind the overriding goal of treatment plan fulfillment and diagnosis verification, which impacts the direction taken between patient and therapist.

Ironically, the popularity of this model is only partially based on scientific validity. The assumption made is that it will lead experts to the closest diagnosis for what is ailing patients. Whether admitted or not, another reason for its success may be in how easily it coincides with a business model of order and cost-effectiveness (Jacob and Patel 2014). Insurance companies, Big Pharma, managed care facilities, and others share business model thinking where it makes more money continuing medical procedures than expecting a cure. Where insurance companies can control what is acceptable or unacceptable for reimbursement. Where managed care facilities can control number of visits and prices for these visits. Unfortunately, at least in my opinion, talk therapy shares a less understood role in this type of practice. These companies or agencies base success on symptom reduction that can be proven, where free-flowing dialogue and the meaning behind a patient's personal story may not be understood or valued.

By comparison, more experiential thinkers in mental health lend themselves to a different set of values where the person in therapy is the focal point of any success or failure in the therapy experience. This includes numerous types of therapy, but for this book, phenomenological and trauma-informed care therapy will be the focus. In both, growth and change become more efficient than symptom reduction. Where becoming aware of one's meaningful stories become more valued than one's unusual behavior. In contrast to a more medical model orientation are those therapists who want to know the experiences of people from many different avenues of meaning. Those areas which define identity as a whole person and the trauma they have gone through including their beliefs, thoughts, feelings, behaviors, and the climate in which they experience mental suffering in their lives. All of these leading to how clients see themselves, specifically their identity. This form of therapy requires an alternative set of skills based on such characteristics as attuned connections, intuition, insight, empathy, selfless acts, and an understanding of hope for future experiences (Ladd 2018).[1] The goal is not necessarily symptom reduction but a connection, a bond between therapist and client, so a free-flowing form of dialogue can help create an alliance between them. In this form of therapy, new avenues of meaning emanating from the dialogue become the focus in order to create hope and to actualize new possibilities for future growth and change (Larsen, Edey, and Lemay 2012).

In more experiential thought, the main instrument used is *dialogue* between therapist and client. Psychopharmacology issues, therapy techniques, and collection of data are not dismissed but are viewed as adjunct concerns to the main goal of creating an ongoing dialogue (Ladd and Churchill 2012). This leads to the importance of an experiential form of treatment and a medical model form of treatment being different in actual practice. Medical model practice is based on finding a diagnosis and the reduction of symptoms. In experiential thinking, there needs to be an ongoing dialogue based on a therapeutic alliance or in trauma-informed care the establishment of safety, in either case, leading to client healing. Both are directed so possibilities for healing can emerge, and hope is created for the future. However, from this less pathological and more positive perspective, if a client is in severe crisis, reducing client symptoms, such as the use of psychotropic drugs, may be involved in clearing a pathway for strong and meaningful collaboration between client and therapist. However, this is a secondary goal to having a strong therapeutic relationship and suppling safety for the client. From medical model thinking if symptoms are reduced then the ultimate goal is achieved. Yet, sometimes only focusing on symptoms reduction can corrupt an understanding of a patient's experiences, leading to a corruption of the healing process.

The same holds true for therapy techniques. When therapy techniques are used as an intervention tool to test out a diagnosis and treatment plan, the shelf life for such procedures is limited unless the client develops some form of ownership of these techniques—no matter how strong the statistical reliability and validity may be of the technique. Techniques may hold meaning for the therapist but not necessarily for the client unless they own them. In more experiential thinking the dialogue between client and therapist may take them to a point in the dialogue where ownership over a therapy technique can be helpful. At this point, the technique finds meaning as a part of the ongoing dialogue that seeks out new possibilities and new hopes for personal growth and change. Experiential thinking believes the client is the unrecognized expert when considering meaningful experiences in a client's life (Ladd and Churchill 2012). This is a major shift from an expert-centered empirical thinking to a more experiential practice where therapy techniques and psychotropic drugs become adjunct activities to the ongoing dialogue between client and therapist.

Let us now look at a few more comparisons as a preview for the upcoming chapters:

- *Why is the thinking in these models basically different?*

A medical model belief is in *knowledge* that must pass statistical reliability and validity as found in the DSM5 and other documents (Bien 2006). It is an accumulation of knowledge that gives credence to mental health diagnoses, treatment plans, and insurance reimbursement. Unfortunately, talking about client experiences does little in helping to validate this thinking, making it a less valuable enterprise in the medical model system. The empirical thinking in the medical model views *scientific truth* by emphasizing an attitude that limits the acceptance of only a certain type of knowledge. If it cannot be validated statistically through a reductionistic, natural scientific empirical formula then it loses much of its importance.

Experiential thinking bases beliefs on a view of getting to each client's individual truth by following the *wisdom* found in the dialogue between client and therapist (Buber 2014). It makes the claim that getting to *each client's truth* will emerge from a client's painful experiences when a meaningful dialogue takes place between client and therapist—both parties adding something to this perceived truth. The goal is to create hope and possibilities for the future, which has little to do with statistical probability but a great deal to do with what practically works. This model does not make the claim that unless one can prove reliability or validity in the ongoing dialogue, it will lose its importance. Effectiveness is a major goal over efficacy. The essence and importance of therapy from this approach is based on the belief that both client and therapist possess a certain unique wisdom based on past experiences, and for the therapist, the recognition of patterns observed within his or her former clients, or through the therapist's own experiences. Through these experiential patterns during meaningful dialogue the belief is that it will alleviate pain, restructure purpose and meaning, and possibly changing one's identity (Ladd 2018).

- *Which way of thinking is more efficient?*[2]

Empirical, medical model thinking will always be more orderly than experiential thinking. It is based on controlling the outcome centered around a preconceived diagnosis, so each step in the process including talk therapy follows predetermined procedures. Such thinking must show a certain order that can have a direct effect on the predetermined outcome. It is a rule-based method of thinking that is geared toward reducing a patient's mental health symptoms. It constantly creates order to focus on reducing patient symptoms. Yet, is this an *efficient* method for solving patient problems?

Collaborative, experiential thinking avoids the mythology of inflexible structured procedures in an ever-changing world, in order to become accurate or efficient in therapy. It is through the unpredictable, free-flowing dialogue where insightful meaning emerges, making this form of thinking more efficient when pursuing and working through a client's personal experiences. In experiential thinking, efficiency is derived from basing success on the accuracy of personal experiences, and not basing efficiency on the statistical analysis of many different client symptoms. One cannot assume that procedures based on statistics which create order are also more efficient, especially when one considers that most of the order is grounded in the business of mental health and not necessarily in the unique experiences of any given client. Sometimes this form of thinking develops complex and efficacious solutions yet may misunderstand the actual problem.

- *How do you measure the importance of knowledge versus wisdom in therapy?*

Empirical medical model thinking is a knowledge-based process that makes calculated decisions regarding the patient's symptoms based on statistical probability. An experiential form of thinking is a wisdom-based process that makes intuitive decisions by immersing both client and therapist into a dialogue surrounding client problems, until both intuitively have insights based on an emerging understanding of the problem (Ladd 2018).

Wisdom is obtained by the constant experiences of the therapist working with any given pattern of pain in a repetitive manner, or from personal experiences of pain such as found in Vietnam War veterans helping Iraqi and Afghani veterans with post-traumatic stress disorder (PTSD). By looking for the unique essences and nuances in client experiences, over time patterns in therapy such as anxiety and depression become familiar in the mind of the therapist (Gladwell 2007). (It is one thing to know something. It is another to wisely know your way around something.) Or, from the constant experiences of pain and suffering from the client, who holds a certain wisdom about their experiences by living it 24/7. However, anxiety or depression may be too close to the client's problems, and therefore he or she lacks wisdom in how to resolve these experiences. Through these intimate forms of collaboration called dialogue between client and therapist, wisdom emerges in a more efficient process. The experiential thinker believes that dialogue will bring us closer to accuracy through the wisdom of experience regarding this one unique client, as opposed to making hypotheses based on a statistical analysis of knowledge based on many clients. The common denominator in a medical model analysis of knowledge is focus only on those characteristics that can be validated statistically at the expense of personal nuances that may be critical in defining each client's suffering. Medical model thinking leads to gathering knowledge to *control* the outcome of therapy by a comparison of one patient's truth to other patients' truths as found in DSM5.

Experiential thinking leads to gathering wisdom through the therapist and client by integration of the dialogue between them (Siegel 2016). The combination of the client's shared experience and the therapist's professional experience with any given dysfunctional pattern or account of a traumatic story is the baseline for acquiring personal truth that is relevant for each client (Ladd and Churchill 2012). The idea of making experiences accountable through reliability and validity standards, as found in the DSM, is to have the "many speak for the one" eliminating unique experiences that clients go through.

In experiential thinking trusting the ability to talk through a problem becomes more valuable by forming a therapeutic alliance and revealing the partnership of shared experiences where both sides will be telling each other the indispensable nuances of the problem as they see it. The accuracy found in the dialogue replaces the diagnoses found in the DSM. One is based on statistics while the other is based on the wisdom found in shared experiences.

- *What is the ultimate goal of a medical model thinking versus an experiential model of thinking?*

The ultimate goal of medical model thinking is to provide relief for the patient. This is accomplished by symptoms reduction and symptom maintenance. It is geared around relief for patient suffering. It may be why psychotropic drugs play such a major role in this process, and why talk therapy seems to play an adjunct or secondary role. In contrast, the ultimate goal of experiential thinking is to provide future meaningful possibilities and hope regarding how a client feels, what they think, how they act, what they believe, and how they see themselves. The concept of healing the whole person is in line with what the neurobiologists would call obtaining balance in all these areas through mindful integration (Siegel 2010). Carl Rogers would call it congruence (Rogers 2003). I am calling it a sense of balance in everyday living. Sometimes relieving symptoms becomes important, and sometimes it is not enough in the healing process.

- *How does medical model thinking and experiential model thinking deal with suffering?*

Medical model thinking is indiscriminate about patient suffering when it comes to mental health. Its purpose is to relieve all suffering that is connected to disorders. Symptoms reduction has remained from the beginning, the major activity that takes place in this form of mental health—which may or may not include talk therapy. In contrast, experiential thinking separates unnecessary suffering from necessary suffering. Unnecessary suffering is any experience that, whether biological or psychological, interferes with the client and therapist discovering meaning and purpose in the client's future. Sometimes psychotropic drugs may be called for in severely disabled clients, who are struggling with finding meaning but become distracted by their emotional pain. However, there are many experiential techniques, such as mindfulness, EMDR, and others, that can take the place of this medical model thinking.

Experiential thinking also understands necessary suffering such as found in grieving, loss, trauma, and any number of experiences that can be worked through rather than accepted as a disorder. Experiential thought encourages a certain wisdom in working through one's suffering, rather than relieving it. Such characteristics such as resilience, motivation, flexibility, and grit can be the results of necessary suffering and integrate well into thinkers who promote a more positive approach to mental health. Regarding ways to think about suffering, a medical model's symptom reduction goal does not necessarily distinguish between necessary and unnecessary suffering (Ladd and Churchill 2012). It treats most suffering the same by trying to reduce it. The sophistication of a phenomenological view of suffering realizes that some suffering is necessary for many different reasons such as positive mood, flexibility, confidence, and so on. It realizes that in the course of a client's experiences some necessary suffering may hold valuable meaning and may even create wisdom that ultimately changes her or his view of themselves.

THE PRACTICE OF EXPERIENTIAL THERAPY

At this point, the struggle over ownership of therapy seems determined more by mental health culture than by what may be best for the client/patient. Therapy being a part of a medical model, where the talking is surrounded by a diagnosis and treatment plan, certainly benefits the professional. It is a neat package that is orderly and can be accounted for by the business of mental health. The elusive meaning behind a free-flowing dialogue between client and therapist based on a therapeutic alliance or the experience of safety, where intuition and insight become as important as statistical probability, seems a higher order of treatment for the client.

Unfortunately, we have not gotten to the point where the benefits of both ways of thinking are recognized and used to help patient/clients. In crisis situations, or when a patient is not in a position to share personal meaning with a therapist, it would be naive to rule out medical model thinking when relief will help certain patients. However, the experiential thinkers in trauma-informed care help in creating safety for the same reasons as prescribing psychotropic drugs. This includes many different types of disorders from anxiety to schizophrenia. Relief from symptoms does seem a human way of helping these people. Yet, when it comes to helping client/patients become stronger by finding meaning and purpose in their lives, an experiential form of thinking helps anxious people as well as schizophrenic people to live a more fulfilled life of hope and possibilities (Cheung 2013).

In the field of mental health, experiential thinking can get lost in the restrictions found in a more empirically based medical model, which seems to dominate most of the mental health practiced in the United States. Yet, there are those thinking professionals in the mental health system that believe symptom reduction and symptom maintenance only address part of the problem regarding the welfare of clients and patients (Lake 2017). The fundamental reason for writing this book is to help define what *is* an experiential therapist, how do they think, and how can this way of thinking assimilate into the mental health industry. For example, the recent COVID-19 outbreak may eventually have a dramatic impact on the future of mental health culture.

Therefore, it may be important in these troubled times for both models to put aside their ideological differences and realize that neither way of thinking should be given priority over the other. Priority may be best served in service to the mental health profession within the culture where it is practiced. Along with a consideration of the empathy found in successful mental health patient/client relationships, a more sophisticated manner of thinking may prevail from the impact of a prevailing worldwide pandemic. It is important not to forget that thinking from a culture in transition, as now being experienced, may have precedence over both ideological thinking where the politics of how to treat mental suffering may not end up being the defining factor in future mental health practice. So, who will own mental health practice in the future world of mental health? It appears to me that having the flexibility to look at all options available makes sense in an ever-changing world where experiential thinking is one of the options.

NOTES

1. These themes and others are found in chapters of the book, *The Talk Therapy Revolution: Neuroscience, Phenomenology and Mental Health.* Lanham, MD: Rowman & Littlefield Publisher.

2. The strength of the experiential model is that one can win the cost-effectiveness argument with the evidence. APA published a summary of this evidence a couple of years ago. Strong evidence has been published in JAMA and by Shedler and has come out of Sweden, Germany, and Belgium. There is also a new edition of Bruce Whampold's book on the evidence for the nonspecific factors in effective therapy.

Chapter 3

A Collaboration Attitude versus an Expert Attitude

A certain subtle attitude develops early when becoming a mental health therapist. This attitude is presented in training where the designated program sets the tone for how one thinks and behaves. Usually there are standards to meet, and to achieve them requires an attitude that matches these standards. This attitude is easily understood for psychiatrists who are already familiar with a medical model way of thinking. It also may fit closely with thinking of other programs outside of psychiatry that want to emulate the behavior of psychiatrists (Willis 2018). Yet, there are those professionals who either come from these programs and who are independent thinkers or are part of programs that focus on human development and question the limitations of a medical model point of view. Their view may be more holistic, more person-centered. For these professionals, having an attitude of getting to know clients/patients in a more phenomenological or experiential manner holds great importance. These are choices that deserve attention, especially at the beginning of training where one's attitude leads to one's behavior.

Unknowingly, are those mental health professionals who accept the attitude that is presented to them from the beginning without a clear understanding of the power involved in this underlying point of view? As important as this attitude may be in affecting the lives of clients/patients, it remains a subtle phenomenon that is just there, usually without being spelled out or challenged in a more comprehensive manner. Before learning diagnosis, before learning psychological techniques, before developing treatment plans lies one's attitude when approaching these skills.

Let it be clear. An attitude for practicing in the field of mental health is not grounded in facts, where facts point to something indisputable. Much of what happens in making judgments in mental health, and specifically in therapy, are based on statistical probability (Nemeroff et al. 2013). So, if you wanted a proper attitude for practicing in the field of mental health, it would be beneficial to focus on one's expertise while avoiding a demeanor of being an expert. That also can be said for one's viewpoint regarding psychotropic drugs or therapy techniques. Experts in mental health cannot make the claim that a therapy technique or a psychotropic drug will work. The best that can be said is that "they probably will work."

So, when clients/patients go to medical model professionals looking for an expert to relieve their pain, what can be promised is "maybe I can help" which leads one to possibly considering an alternative choice (Neubauer 2019). One based on a collaborative attitude when facing clients/patients. Granted, there are medical model therapists who are collaborative, making these comments appear trivial unless one considers that some mental health professionals have a mindset based on the "fixed are helping the broken" with patient mental illness. Putting it bluntly, we all are broken in some way when considering our lives and having the possibility of a mental health issue. As said before, as professionals it may be more effective to develop an expertise that one can be proud of accomplishing, rather than having a demeanor of an expert.

Let us consider a different attitude. A more collaborative one in mental health practice that starts out with the notion that "maybe I can help you, with your support." This does not diminish the value placed on psychotropic drugs or specific therapy techniques. It may even emphasize the importance of collaboration between client and therapist when using these drugs and skills in a meaningful way. Especially when a client and therapist include them in a collaborative dialogue during therapy. Such a change in attitude seems more relevant than a twentieth-century, medical model, rules-based system that relies on probability rather than a more twenty-first-century, postmodern, problem-solving model based on collaboration and possibility (Ladd 2013). However, such a collaborative way of thinking may face challenges by the ongoing use of the medical model in mental health.

For instance, it does reflect on the issue of who is in control? When dealing with severe cases of psychosis the expectation may be that the mental health professional requires a certain level of control, and a collaborative attitude may not be as beneficial, yet this point is debatable. The days of the mental health professional being viewed as the indisputable expert are slowly drifting away (Walters 2015). To better understand this, let us consider a comparison between a collaborative and expert attitude in mental health.

The idea of wanting to collaborate begins with working together to create something new in support of a shared vision. The key points in developing this attitude are it is not through individual effort, something new is created, and the glue is the shared vision (Feire et al. 2018). On the other hand, an expert is a person with extensive knowledge or ability based on research, experience, or occupation, and in a particular area of study. This can be an individual effort or the effort of a team of experts who are identified by a certain expertise (Sandell et al. 2007). In mental health, both of these definitions shape the attitude of the therapist from the beginning of training. In the medical model, the therapist bases his or her understanding on gathered knowledge that eventually decides a diagnosis and a treatment plan, both requiring a certain expertise. These are acquired either academically or experientially, usually through a standardized set of procedures that fit the mental health medical model.

There is an expectation that the therapist has the knowledge to make judgments and decisions that benefit their patients, and many patients in this system have a similar attitude and expect the therapist to have the answers, and to prescribe the solutions. This point of view applies to most professionals in the care of people's health. You do not go to a dentist with an understanding that you will be co-extractor of a tooth or a doctor where she or he asks you to reset your broken leg. The expectations are clear. The professional is the expert, and the patient is the recipient of this expertise.

In mental health, this belief is not so clear, either with the therapist or sometimes with the client. It is correct that a mental health therapist needs knowledge and experience in order to be effective, yet the experience needed can also lie in the hands of the client. They live their suffering 24/7, and even though they may lack the knowledge or expertise to overcome their suffering, they certainly feel it, think it, behave accordingly to it, and have an attitude about it.

The experiential therapist whether having a background in phenomenology or trauma-informed care considers the clients perspective and involvement in the experience of suffering and takes on a more collaborative attitude. This is based on the premise that therapy should not be an individual effort but a collaborative one. An experiential therapist enters therapy as someone who can collaborate with clients in a safe and meaningful way. While an expert attitude toward therapy is based on predetermined assumptions, an experiential attitude limits these assumptions. Both enter the profession with a belief system they consider valid and accurate. The expert attitude begins therapy with a general collection of data to back up one's expertise in forming a diagnosis and treatment plan. Conversely, the collaborative attitude believes there is an impediment to therapy by starting with a series of predetermined assumptions. It advocates for a free-flowing dialogue based on the client's experiences, and one can find value in both points of view. Unfortunately, the mental health profession has fallen behind other disciplines such as in the law where some problems need to be litigated while others can be mediated (Mnookin 1998). Or, in business where some decisions are made from the top down while others come from the bottom up (Johnson 2018).

In mental health, there is a reliance on the natural scientific method that tends to subjugate more experiential methods as "tack on" to a higher empirical standard. However, this does not discount the legitimacy of a collaborative model of psychological assessment. Constance Fischer's classic book, *Individualizing Psychological Assessment*, which appeared over thirty years ago has become increasingly mainstream over the decades (Fischer 1994). Fischer was a pioneer in the development of phenomenological clinical psychological assessment at the American home of the movement, Duquesne University.

However, for the time being, let us treat both attitudes with equality. As stated previously, an expert attitude requires structured plans that are agreed upon before therapy, and a collaborative attitude believes less in structured plans. From a collaborative viewpoint, the interactions are marked by moment-to-moment adjustments, in which therapists base their decisions on the flow of the conversation centered around the particular clients' meaningful stories, rather than empirically driven analysis. The expert attitude is based on predetermined goals, while the collaborative attitude is based on characteristics of the particular experiences that determine the next move in collaboration with the client.

So, which is more valuable: the attitude of the medical model therapist, the beliefs held by the experiential therapist, or can both be valuable? It would be hard to argue that with severe mental disorders such as schizophrenia, the skills of an expert can be valuable, especially when it involves psychopharmacology. Yet, studies suggest that therapists who build on their experiences have a more flexible attitude, and they cope better with more complex conditions and severe problems, and are able to form more complex, nuanced personal connections than colleagues who do not build on their experiences (Collard 2018). A collaborative attitude toward therapy puts value in former experiences of the therapist and uses these experiences to build an expertise with clients, rather than an expertise that is formulated around such manuals as the DSM 5. Yet, trying to determine the attitude of individual therapists may be a losing proposition. In all fairness, it is possible to follow a strict medical model and still use a semi-experiential model to connect with clients.

Mental health may need to decide whether there is room for alternative models within each therapist's professional belief system. Can having a more balanced perspective between expertise and collaboration be allowed to practice in our present mental health system? Can a professional therapist have a philosophy that includes both models and use them when it seems appropriate?

These questions become relevant when dealing with the current state of mental health where insurance companies and Big Pharma indirectly influence the attitudes of therapists. Sometimes the pressures of the workplace make subtle demands on mental health professionals to follow procedures not necessarily based on ideology or preference but based on economics where insurance reimbursement and Big Pharma set the tone in mental health (Ladd 2018). Sometimes professionals will make the comment, "This is what I have to do, not what I want to do." Unfortunately, compliance in one's profession caused by outsiders may not be a motivating factor for either the client or the professional. Some would argue that having an attitude where a therapist must conform to outside institutions such as insurance or Big Pharma may be a practice in mediocrity, reinforced through compliance.

CASE STUDY

Joan reported to her mental health provider about having continued negative experiences that were changing the way she viewed herself. She stated that over time she was becoming increasingly isolated and feeling worthless. She told her provider how shocked she was by these changes, because this was not the way she perceived her life. She also reported that the stress of life led to abusing alcohol and reported that a subtle feeling of doing something wrong permeated her emotions. Joan stated that a lack of motivation was stirring feelings of guilt leading to more worthless feelings. She also described a sense of loss by going through this experience. It was reported that some of her loss was due to loss of interest, loss of appetite, loss of motivation, and loss of sleep. She felt a failure for being unsuccessful in coping with this problem (Ladd and Churchill 2012).

A Expert Attitude

The following is an example of Joan's case study during her sessions at a mental health clinic. It is what *might happen* to anyone caught up in life's traumas. For now, let us try to produce a reasonable description using a medical model format in approaching Joan's problems.

After the initial intake, the person in charge worked from a position that enough symptoms existed to make a hypothesis that Joan may be suffering from some form of depression. This information was passed on to a psychiatrist, who used a checklist to further assess Joan during an evaluation session. The psychiatrist checked off some of the cluster of symptoms found in the DSM for depression, namely feelings of worthlessness, sleep disturbance, feelings of isolation, appetite disturbance, and guilt. The psychiatrist also questioned her on how long these symptoms were present and determined they lasted for an appropriate amount of time to qualify as a disorder. The psychiatrist also observed such issues as non-expressive mood, cloths being ruffled, and other behavioral gestures lacking the effect of someone who is normally engaged in the world.

Later, at a team meeting the psychiatrist determined that Joan was suffering from the mood disorder, depression, and that an entry-level dose of Prozac seemed appropriate. From the therapists in the team meeting, a treatment plan was developing that would include some form of CBT. A mental health therapist would be assigned to assist Joan in fulfilling the treatment plan, especially regarding feelings of guilt, isolation, sleep disturbances, and appetite.

After a few sessions with Joan, her therapist eventually pointed out Joan's symptoms, and the importance of changing one's irrational thoughts. When the therapist felt Joan grasped the concept of CBT, they changed direction to work on her sleeping patterns, feelings of guilt, isolation, and appetite. As one issue on the treatment plan was completed, the therapist moved on to the next, always checking on how she was responding to the prescribed Prozac. Joan also was asked to keep a diary of her progress, which was shared by the therapist at each treatment meeting. After twelve visits, the treatment team decided that she had completed therapy, and the decision was made for Joan to spend the next few sessions getting closure on her issues. (Her insurance plan would allow up to fourteen sessions.) The psychiatrist also recommended she continue with Prozac for the next eighteen months based on her reporting feelings of calmness.

The medical model treatment regarding Joan in this case study is not the "Cookbook" method for all people who are feeling this way. Yet, enough of Joan's feelings fit with the guidelines in the DSM to be considered a high probability that Joan suffered from depression. The therapy team worked from the attitude of knowing what was wrong based on the collective information given, and by following a medical model format. It was from an expert attitude and the knowledge found in the DSM where conclusions were made early on that Joan had symptoms of depression. Many psychiatrists, and other medical model loyalists, see themselves as experts, and the DSM is the agreed-upon arbitrator of conclusions, bolstering an attitude of being knowledgeable professionals in mental health. Medical model hospitals and clinics have a similar attitude regarding what is being presented in this case study, and most training programs subtly infer the same attitude (Fitcher 2019).[1]

What if mental health professionals viewed themselves not as experts but as collaborators? Would they be more inclined to have Joan describe her experiences and the meaning behind them? Would this collaboration help the diagnosis and treatment plan align with Joan's experiences? Would a more bio/psycho/social medical model differ from a strict medical model, even though it followed a predetermined diagnosis and treatment plan? Or, would it be beneficial both for the client/patient and the therapist to work from an attitude of collaboration until the true meaning of her experiences were revealed?

A Collaboration Attitude

The following is what happened to Joan during her 2012 *real-life* sessions at a clinic that allowed for a more phenomenological perspective. The clinic desired a more collaborative attitude while working within the boundaries of a medical model. One might say they were working from an experiential/medical model. The clinic in question tried to balance the needs of the present medical model culture with the attitudes of therapists who worked in the clinic. This real-life case study is being presented for those who have to follow a medical model, yet prefer a more collaborative point of view in actual practice.

From the beginning of Joan's entrance into the mental health clinic, the position of the staff was positive and engaging. She was told that an initial interview would take place where her thoughts and feelings were an important part of how the therapy would proceed. It was described as a motivational interview where more than descriptive information could be shared. Where the point of view of the client was considered a meaningful part of what took place. During the interview it became clear that some symptoms described by Joan fit within the boundaries of clinical depression. Yet, other concerns were added by Joan regarding her past and present experiences. She was concerned about how isolated she felt, how the feeling of rejection caused her a considerable amount of pain and relieving it by drinking excessive amounts of alcohol was not working.

From a psychiatric perspective, there was enough evidence to approach the psychiatrist working on staff, who could have prescribed some form of antidepressant. This did not happen based on two perspectives: (1) the therapist involved did not view Joan as someone who was in severe crisis and who would have trouble sharing her experiences, and (2) Joan did not want to take psychotropic drugs, at that time. Later at a team meeting, the psychiatrist who met with Joan collaborated with her therapist and also considered Joan's perspective for not using psychotropic drugs. The psychiatrist concluded that Joan's case should be reviewed regarding drugs after a therapeutic alliance was formed between Joan and the therapist.

The treatment plan for this clinic was not necessarily a plan but more of an attitude. It was based on the importance of a therapeutic alliance being formed before considering any future plans. For the next four sessions, Joan slowly revealed some of the experiences that caused her symptoms of depression. She described a pattern of isolation, rejection, and pain based on the abandonment of her one true love many years before. From that time on, she decided not to risk a deep relationship, ever again. As the alliance was formed by Joan and the therapist, it was revealed that her experiences were pointing toward a pattern of loneliness, combined with some symptoms of depression. She shared how her isolation added to her feelings of rejection which eventually ended in a hollow and empty feeling of pain. Finally, after a strong alliance was formed, she realized her excessive drinking was an attempt to relieve the pain, yet it was only temporary until the isolation again set in.

At a team meeting, after the alliance with Joan was fully formed, the therapist represented Joan's experiences to the staff after collaborating with Joan on what the therapist would share.

For insurance purposes and based on depression manifesting itself in her experiences, the psychiatrist made a diagnosis based on the mood disorder, depression. For the therapist and Joan, a different collaborative dialogue became the focus of attention. They agreed to face her loneliness head on. (As a sidenote, the idea of using psychotropic drugs in this case became irrelevant.) In order to work through her loneliness, both the therapist and Joan agreed that relieving the pain through alcohol or antidepressants might not be the correct avenue to follow. She agreed to test the courage in working through her pain instead of reducing it and to risk reconnecting with others in the outside world.

What follows in Joan's case study will take too long to describe regarding the accomplishments made in her remaining sessions. However, all the sessions focused around overcoming Joan's loneliness, and Joan did recover and began reconnecting in meaningful relationships. (In later chapters the skills and procedures used in a more phenomenological model will be presented. For now, let it be stated that in Joan's case study, all the skills were accomplished in collaboration between the client and therapist.)

DISCUSSION

In the above collaborative method for resolving Joan's problems could be viewed as invalid and unreliable from a classic medical model perspective. The question one might ask, "How could this be possible?" The answer may be found in an expert attitude that subtly puts pressure on the therapist to unwittingly rely on the knowledge from the DSM, in order to be valid. It could be argued that loneliness found in Joan's case study cannot be authenticated by knowledge found in the DSM. Loneliness may be a life experience, but it is not a disorder, even though at the present time there appears to be an epidemic of loneliness. The preference is still to emphasize the mood disorder of depression. Thus, to focus on loneliness is to lose what can be empirically proven as valid, namely depression. Can a therapist working from a classic medical model even consider a diagnosis of loneliness and devote most of therapy to that end? Or, are client experiences only recognized if they are found in a cluster of symptoms in a book based on statistical probability? For those who believe this and have an expert attitude, may find this collaborative example intriguing but not within the realm of medical model procedures. They may be drawn to follow the DSM rather than client experiences.

An expert attitude in a medical model relies on empirical values over experiential values. If you cannot prove your case empirically, it loses its value. A collaborative attitude in an experiential model relies on experiential values before considering empirical values, making a case for a different set of practices during therapy. In this approach, the therapist is trying to capture the meaning within a client's experiences, or the therapy loses its value. In the above comparison, the medical model experts proved their case by listing Joan's symptoms and time line for depression as found in the probability factors inside the DSM. All the symptoms in the DSM had to be reliable and valid according to the statistical measurements that empower this document.

Conversely, an experiential model with a more collaborative attitude is looking for accuracy within the client's experiences, which may shift the focus away from a psychiatric evaluation. Even though a medical model diagnosis of depression did exist, it was not at the heart of the meaningful experiences that Joan was encountering. The actual meaning behind her depression and suffering was a pattern of loneliness that slowly unfolded as the collaboration between client and therapist moved toward establishing a therapeutic alliance. From this perspective, the expert conclusion from the medical model therapists was helpful but not as conclusive as the powerful sense of loneliness that Joan was experiencing in collaboration with her therapist.

Continuing in this review, an expert attitude also can be viewed in how precise the diagnosis fits the criteria in the DSM. Compared this to a collaboration attitude based on being comprehensive but not necessarily needing precision. The medical model diagnosis for Joan was formulated on the precision demonstrated in the rules and guidelines found in the DSM. For the most part, this precision was all that was needed to develop a diagnosis and treatment plan. The experiential diagnosis for Joan was formulated from a more comprehensive view. Joan's loneliness was demonstrated in a pattern depicting loneliness that was recognizable to her, that helped in recognizing her personal experience with loneliness. It was not statistically precise but comprehensive enough to capture the meaningful essence of the loneliness phenomenon. It was demonstrated by the ongoing changes based on the revelation of new and meaningful experiences regarding Joan's suffering through her loneliness. In a medical model, the diagnosis was fulfilled by the precise number of symptoms that rendered the diagnosis of depression. In the experiential model, the diagnosis kept changing based on the collaboration between Joan and her therapist. In establishing an alliance, Joan felt comfortable enough to finally tell the story behind her loneliness. The collaboration between client and therapist captured in therapy the comprehensive and essential meaning of how loneliness was wrecking her life.

In many ways, it also may come to what kind of attitude does one use in the collection of data? A medical model expert attitude is looking for statistical data that can hold a probability of success. That is why the DSM is based not on personal patterns of experience but on *statistical data* based on probability. If you cannot find it in the DSM or some other empirical measurement, it may be the data remains unreliable and short of valid. An experiential collaborative attitude is looking for *meaning-based data* that reflect a client's unique life experiences. Experiential data is based more on patterns of experience that capture any given phenomenon, not statistics. For example, in the case study, the collaboration between Joan and her therapist slowly moved the collaborative dialogue toward a pattern that coincided more with loneliness than depression. Isolation, rejection, pain, working through pain, risking, reconnecting with the outside world, all became meaningful stages in her experience. The pattern of loneliness had a purpose and meaning to be "worked through" rather than only reduced to symptoms, and the experiential diagnosis reflects what she was working through more than what label may define her as a person (figure 3.1).

The primitive pattern visualized in figure 3.1 is not based on facts nor is it based on probability. It is based on trying to understand Joan's experience of loneliness by creating possibilities for change. It is not a pattern based on empirical precision but one based on a more comprehensive set of recognizable possibilities for ongoing dialogue in therapy. Out of collaboration between client and therapist can emerge creative possibilities while discussing the pattern above. However, this is but one method for pointing out patterns of experience. The more important point is that a climate of collaboration makes such patterns possible, whether they are presented visually, vocally, or emotionally.

The medical model culture in mental health makes it difficult to visualize even small changes in procedures, let alone a cultural revolution that would expand expertise to include collaboration—though I have strongly advocated for this to happen (Ladd 2018). What the case study does reveal

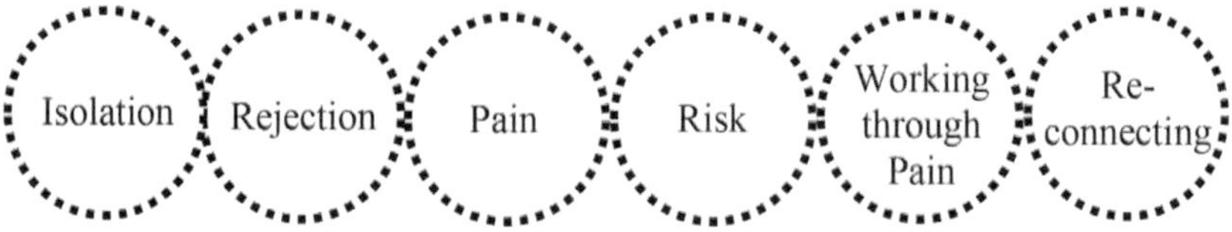

Figure 3.1 Collaborative Pattern of Loneliness for Joan.

is collaboration combined with expertise that brings us closer to helping our clients/patients both empirically and experientially.

The above discussion is not a battle over which model wins the day. It is an observation that each case coming before those practicing in the mental health industry might consider expanding their attitudes. By developing more sophistication, instead of unknowingly practicing without understanding their personal attitudes toward mental health. The creative energy that can be found in working as a therapist can expand to include not only client symptoms but also client experiences. There is a time and place for having an expert or collaborative attitude in therapy, but it should not depend on an inflexible set of guidelines that does not necessarily direct a therapist to the actual experiences of patients. Rather, it directs them to a book filled with statistical probabilities. It may be more important to critically think through a problem than define it by the DSM. That having flexibility in procedures that complement actual experiences is more valuable than having experience awkwardly fit into standardized procedures. Under these conditions, a collaborative attitude can function. Even within the walls of a medical model there may be room for an experiential therapist.

NOTE

1. Additional examples of phenomenological assessment can be found in Peter Ladd. 1974. *The Phenomenological Experience of Fear.* San Diego, CA: U.S. International University (Thesis) and Peter Ladd. 1976. *Resentment of Authority from a Phenomenological Approach.* San Diego, CA: U.S. International University (Dissertation).

Chapter 4

Wisdom versus Knowledge

We[1] retain knowledge, but we obtain wisdom (Elberty 2019). Knowledge is something that we retain and collect. In mental health, it is collected, retained, and normalized and marks the beginning stage in becoming a mental health therapist. Most of it is stored in the hippocampus, the limbic region of the brain, and without it, we remain in the dark and unaware of our options or choices. In mental health and especially in mental health therapy, years may be spent retaining knowledge that hopefully will make a professional aware of relevant practices in therapy. It is the retention of knowledge that acts as a foundation for making calculated decisions during the course of a mental health career. When working with client/patients, knowledge from mental health education combined with the compilation of other expert knowledge, for example, knowledge from the DSM, makes a therapist credible and certified as a legitimate professional.

As important as retained knowledge may be for a mental health therapist, there is no guarantee that she or he will gain the wisdom to use it. Wisdom is not rooted in retention. It is obtained through experience and education that one uses in the world. In mental health therapy, wisdom develops in different ways. One example is to use the knowledge learned and fine-tune it through practice. Another is to practice what is successful while working with clients. Where a therapist obtains certain experiences of success that qualify as wisdom. For example, by successfully forming a therapeutic alliance over and over again, a therapist may intuitively develop a pattern of wisdom that can be employed with different clients when creating such an alliance. It is not retained knowledge that creates wisdom, though retaining knowledge from education does help in awareness. More important for the therapist is the successful practice of retained knowledge or obtained successful experiences that have the potential for creating wisdom. When wisdom is achieved a neurological/phenomenological experience happens both simultaneously in the therapist's brain and in the therapist's world. Neurologically and phenomenologically a pattern develops that recognizes, for example, from the limbic region of the brain, "Now is the time to address that troubled gesture just made by the client." Wisdom goes beyond retaining knowledge. It also improves within the therapist a sense of purpose and timing, and the ability to act directly in the present moment.

Unlike retained knowledge, wisdom is more complicated than using the logic center found in the cerebral cortex, which is then stored in the hippocampus or memory center. Wisdom becomes deeply influenced by the limbic portion in our emotional center of the brain and especially the amygdala, the part of the brain that reacts to prelogical awareness (Zhu 2018). The emphasis on the emotional centers found in the limbic region makes wisdom more intuitive than logical (Schwartz 2017). The formation of wisdom is through the instincts of the therapist that develop intuitively into insightful patterns at any given moment in therapy. These patterns are subconsciously understood both experientially and neurologically. They may pop out when working with clients through valuable insights, not based on retained knowledge but based on obtained wisdom (Ladd 2018).

The reliance on instincts creates the phenomenon of intuition leading to "aha moments" or insights during therapy. Yet, this does not fully describe why wisdom may be more dynamic than retained knowledge in the actual practice of mental health therapy. Therapists also obtain wisdom by making mistakes. If the first time you put your hand on a hot stove, you hopefully have the wisdom not to put it there again. Your experience through making a mistake adds to your wisdom, unless you have learned nothing from your experience and make the same mistake twice. (One of the issues in mental health therapy are those clients who continue to make the same mistakes over and over again.) In this example, wisdom has little to do with retained knowledge; however, the realization of making mistakes holds the same configurations in the brain that form patterns of success in the outside world, and to a wise therapist both are valuable, one by relying on past successes and the other choosing not to make the same mistake twice (Stosny 2014).

Experientially, both success and failure offer the therapist a different form of knowledge described as *personal tacit knowledge* when working with clients—not on logical calculations but on intuitive insights based on wisdom (Polanyi 1974). Metaphorically speaking, small particles of unconscious tacit knowledge will envelop and attach to the explicit conscious knowledge shared between therapist and client, creating nuances that become a major contributor to the wisdom shared between them (more in chapter 8).

However, for now let me give an example. A mental health graduate student was working with a teenage boy. The client had come across his father's suicide, and now the graduate student was struggling with reaching the boy in counseling. He asked me to observe him at the next meeting. As I watched, he was doing effectively most of what we were teaching in our program but with no success. He asked me to intervene. I did so, and after about twenty minutes the boy broke down and shared his true feelings. Later the student asked, "You did exactly what I tried to do, so I do not understand my outcome." I tried to explain about the small particles of tacit knowledge coming from my unconscious that surrounded my explicit conscious knowledge and counseling skills. I believe that my explanation was unsuccessful. A few years later he e-mailed me and said, "I now get it. My procedures got in the way of my wisdom." I e-mailed him back, "Congratulations, you have discovered what I believe is the hardest lesson in becoming a mental health counselor namely, using your personal knowledge to help people." As Polanyi would say, "We know more than we can tell" (1974).

Also, this form of therapy will be grounded in a form of emotional intelligence (EI) not in a cognitive intellect (Goleman 2005). This alone should raise wisdom to an equally important practice in mental health therapy, as calculating a diagnosis and creating a treatment plan. It should be considered valuable within the structure of mental health culture. It should make intuition and tacit knowledge as important as calculations, or more specifically diagnosing through statistical probability. It should make insight deriving from unconscious tacit knowledge important as relying on a cluster of symptoms to frame the reality around any given patient/client. *It should make obtained wisdom as important as retained knowledge.*

So, why has the field of mental health drawn its eyes away from the wisdom found in using one's personal tacit knowledge and experience and replaced them with a more standardized view of reality as found in the DSM? In answering the question of "why," I refer you to a book by Scholl and Hansen called *Postmodern Perspectives on Contemporary Counseling Issues* (2018) for a more in-depth understanding of this issue where politics and power appear more economic than ideological.

For some experientially oriented therapists this realization may stand out dramatically. They may appreciate the knowledge from logical and empirical sources such as the DSM 5 but seek out the use of wisdom found in their professional experiences using meaningful successes and failures in their development. Yet, others may abandon their personal tacit knowledge and experiences by getting lost in the perceived conundrum inherent in medical model procedures, or they may practice in the shadows of appearing compliant while treating their brand of therapy as a covert activity.

There seems to be a dichotomy when comparing retained knowledge with obtained wisdom in mental health. The empirical procedures in mental health appear to hold more value than a therapist's personal tacit knowledge and experience, especially when the perceptions by therapist/patient view suffering differently than perceptions from the DSM. Another reason that contemporary medical model culture appears to overlook wisdom is that it is difficult to learn without experience. Retained knowledge is gained through the teachings found in the culture of mental health therapy. The emphasis then lies with experts who can teach how to be an effective therapist. As a profession, it would be difficult to discount the research, techniques, procedures, philosophies, and history that go into retaining knowledge that meet the standards of becoming a credible mental health therapist.

Unfortunately, there is no guarantee the therapists know how to use this retained knowledge if they abandon the tacit personal knowledge that was accumulated over the myriad of experiences in their lives. I believe when clients come to therapy in disarray, broken and confused, they are looking not for retained knowledge but for the obtained wisdom of the therapist. I also believe, each therapist's personal tacit knowledge and experiences belongs to no one else, and that authenticity grounded in personal experiences creates trust in the clients/therapist relationship. Under these circumstances, and especially in experiential thinking, therapy depends on dialogue based on different human experiences, the experiences of the client, and hopefully the wisdom found in the personal tacit knowledge and experiences of the therapist. Healing begins within this dialogue of experiences generated by wisdom-influenced therapy. Ironically, after meaningful human connections are made, the possibility for retained knowledge through standard therapy techniques becomes more of a viable option, a lesson that should be a consideration for strict medical model professionals clinging to natural scientific methodology.

Yet, the value put on the retained explicit knowledge, based on medical model thinking in mental health, leaves little room for personal tacit knowledge or experiences, even when the medical model therapist has obtained a considerable amount of wisdom. They still are bound by the procedures and guidelines included in natural scientific methodology. Subsequently, more resistant experiential therapists may find their wisdom ignored leading to "not what they want to do, but what they have to do through the predetermined protocol inherent in the medical model." This overemphasis on the retained explicit knowledge that qualifies a therapist as a professional may hinder, in real time, one's professional wisdom, unless there is an awareness that both hold equal value.

Let us now apply what often happens in medical model therapy and make a brief comparison with experiential therapy. For the medical model therapist, the collection of knowledge determines the direction taken in therapy. In other words, you have to do what was taught that authorities deem important, within the guidelines of a medical model, or insurance companies, or managed care guidelines. These guidelines or procedures circle around symptoms and labels obtained from the DSM. The knowledge is then applied in a treatment plan.

An experiential therapist relies more on wisdom through personal experiences or personal tacit knowledge. The therapist unconsciously recognizes patterns stored in the brain where particles of this tacit knowledge stick to the intentionality in what is included in the dialogue between client and therapist. Wisdom may involve optimal balance between functions of phylogenetically more primitive brain regions (limbic system) and newer ones (prefrontal cortex) (Meeks and Jeste 2013). In therapy, a client's stories, emotional outbursts, or forgotten memories may trigger these patterns, intuitively directing the therapist toward dialogue filled with insight. This ongoing process and the insights revealed determine the direction taken in therapy. In experiential therapy, the unique experiences of the client create insight—not a predetermined series of calculated decisions before therapy begins. Through dialogue, vital parts of the experiences are revealed to both client and therapist. Neurologically, the brain stores patterns and phenomenologically these patterns become recognizable in the outside world (Ladd 2018). Instinctively, intuitively, and eventually insightfully this combination can turn into a more accurate experience that is grounded in the personal reality of the client.

So, are there skills through retained knowledge found in one's training that increase wisdom in therapy? Sometimes, it is important to keep in mind that wisdom is based on using knowledge not retaining it. Within an acceptance in deciding to be a therapist, the profession itself advocates for "do no harm" and herein lies the wisdom inherent in professionalism when practicing mental health therapy. Some of that professionalism has already been discussed regarding intuition, where wise therapists appear more intuitive, and use it more frequently during therapy. Intuition is a way of perceiving a situation by looking at the whole picture. It incorporates history and looks for broad general patterns. It also contemplates the future. It assesses where the current situation might be going (Gladwell 2007). Why therapists use it more frequently, one finds its basic structure in the idea that *trust has superior accuracy over control* (Ladd 2018). The knowledge retained from medical model therapy is grounded more in controlling the variables for a successful outcome. This explains the focus on collecting information before creating a diagnosis and treatment plan. It also explains why control becomes an important component in remaining an expert, based on retained knowledge during the therapy process.

In comparison, experiential therapists practicing wisdom have a belief system that does not completely rely on retained knowledge based on control. Through intuition they may go beyond it when subtle nuances, concepts, and possibly gestures emerge in the dialogue between client and therapist.

Experiential therapists trust the experience of intuition for its accuracy and on occasions abandon the treatment plans and focus on the meaningful dialogue taking place. The medical model's strong emphasis on standardization and professional procedures sometimes makes this a difficult proposition. However, you will find that many postmodern oriented therapists have the power experienced by using tacit knowledge in their practices through techniques such as narrative therapy, solution-focused therapy, and trauma-informed therapy, just to name a few.

Another set of beliefs and values found when practicing wisdom is the selfless attitude it brings to therapy. The concept of trust is the belief system behind the selfless acts of collaboration, and not necessarily on controlling the therapist's predetermined treatment plan. Neurologically it is the mirror neurons that make an intimate connection between client and therapist (Puder 2019). Experientially, it is the practice of positive regard that keeps the focus on the client (Rogers and Wood 1974). Wisdom promotes selfless acts in therapy that are not found in retained knowledge of the therapist but in the closeness of connection between therapist and client—that subtle but dynamic sense of being attuned to each other's feelings (Ladd 2018). It becomes that visceral connection that conjures up in the therapist's previous experiences that emerge as insight. Unfortunately, it suggests the difficulty when predetermined sets of guidelines and rules are strictly controlling the direction taken during therapy. In present mental health culture, mental health therapists are not trained to value spontaneous selfless acts based on trust. Having a selfless attitude found in wisdom may be too threatening for a model that depends on procedures, fabricated through retained knowledge, and minimized through a need for control.

CASE STUDY

Frank was a child of the 1980s. He grew up in a loving environment and had many opportunities to develop his own mind. Fortunately, this was the case because an inherent speech impediment did not bode well for his early childhood education. So, Frank began to compensate for his lack of academic ability, and his difficulty with social interactions. Instead, he became a keen observer of other people's actions and gestures. He seemed to have an edge over his peers in knowing what was going on in any given situation. Over time, this led to friends and other students seeking out his opinions on problems that seemed to baffle them. Here he could, in a limited amount of words, give his valued opinions. Others liked him and he treated them in an engaging and hospitable way. After years of elocution lessons, his speech impediment began to fade. Some said that he grew out of it, but if the truth be told, he worked himself out of it by depending on both successful and unsuccessful experiences.

During his teenage years, Frank faced many of the same temptations as his friends. Developmentally, he faced the need to experiment with drugs and alcohol. He also faced a need to rebel, and this unfortunately got him in trouble on numerous occasions. His experimentation with drugs and alcohol was brief after watching his friends wreck their lives physically and through others being arrested by law enforcement. Regarding his rebellion, it seemed to shift away from conflicts with parents, teachers, and other authorities to more of a rebellion against society's social system. When entering college, he believed that he could help change the inequalities found in society, until 9/11 influenced his direction entirely.

Believing that an injustice happened to the country, he found himself in the experience of the Iraqi war as a combat soldier. Not being able to speak the language, and not knowing the Iraqi culture, unconsciously forced him to use the same set of skills learned during the early days in school when fighting his speech impediment. He became an observer of human gestures, of certain looks, of specific cultural behaviors, of different tones of voice from the Iraqi people. He also observed some of the same gestures, looks, tones of voice among the soldiers who fought and died around him.

By the time he returned from Iraq, his perception had changed from the experience of killing to one of helping. While continuing his education, psychology became a major curiosity in developing his belief in helping others. Eventually, Frank found himself engaged in a doctoral degree program in clinical psychology where he seemed to flourish in the knowledge obtained from the courses required for the degree. This began to shift during a yearlong internship in a mental hospital where he was responsible for the diagnosis and treatment of people who presented with symptoms of psychosis. Many of the usual procedures were practiced, anywhere from actual diagnosis to shared treatment plan meetings where they reviewed each professional's assigned patients, including the patients of the internship students at the hospital.

During the course of the year, Frank was assigned a patient that, in his opinion, did not fit the diagnosis he was given. He was diagnosed with schizophreniform disorder based on the gibberish that he constantly communicated when talking with professionals, or to anyone else. His lack of hygiene and his disregard for practicing normal social rituals and his withdrawal from family, friends, and social activities all pointed to his diagnosed disorder. Frank made a point in his progress notes that continued to reinforce this diagnosis and was praised by his colleagues for the quality of his descriptions, which matched their views about this patient.

Yet, something was bothering him. His patient, who we will call George, did not have the vacant "shark eyes" prevalent in so many others in his care.

His gestures were erratic yet seemed to point to something more intentional, as though he was looking for a response. His language went something like this, (Frank) "Hi George how are you doing today?" (George) "edital lgli-gook meglobg durnf." Frank would respond, "Thank you George, I am just checking in to see how you are doing." Frank would walk away with two distinct thoughts: George's condition had not changed and intuition told him that something was missing. At a team meeting, Frank shared his concerns but was immediately told that he should stick with the diagnosis and that he was doing an excellent job, especially with this particular case.

The problem with his colleague's conclusions were that over the years Frank had developed a different method of perceiving the world, one might say a method based on successful and unsuccessful experiences grounded in his personal knowledge and experience. One that kept bothering him as he treated George. One day, Frank began talking to George in this manner: (Frank) "pnfgek shrub ldleh demote." With caution and astonishment, George slowly responded with, "jdtsk edcvb pdbhet." Frank positively nodded to him, and with a smile moved on to another patient. Over the course of a month, the same gibberish was heard from both sides of the conversation. Frank's superiors found his behavior erratic and a bit unprofessional. During team meetings there was a combination of disingenuousness and disapproval from his colleagues, yet Frank continued on with his gibberish-focused discourse with George.

One day while sitting on a bench with Frank, George asked, "Can I go to the bathroom?" Frank responded, "Yes, go ahead." It took Frank about two or three minutes to realize that George had asked a question in English. Upon his return, Frank blurted out, "Why are you speaking to me in English?" George's response changed Frank's outlook on mental health therapy from that point moving forward. George said, "I have been through numerous traumas where I was judged and condemned for my behavior. I eventually realized when acting with gibberish and other behaviors, that people would leave me alone." It was at that point where Frank and George had connected and formed a strong therapeutic alliance. Over numerous sessions, George finally asked Frank, "How do I get out of here?" Frank's answer was simple: "Begin to talk in full sentences, and practice impeccable hygiene, and there is a chance that you will leave this institution." The end of the story is that Frank graduated and moved to a job as an assistant professor of psychology a number of months later. However, he had heard that George, indeed, left the hospital, and was on his way to a full recovery.

Eventually, Frank found himself in the position of teaching graduate students about such courses as psychopathology, diagnosis, techniques of therapy, and many other medical model requirements. The difference in his teaching compared to some of his colleagues was his willingness to discuss the power and accuracy that one might find in personal knowledge and experience. Knowledge that developed into a sense of wisdom regarding mental health therapy. He felt that his students at least had a foundation in the value of wisdom, if or when they had an opportunity to practice it. He felt they entered the profession of therapy with more than one perspective based on empiricism, a more experiential perspective fitting a more experiential therapist.

DISCUSSION

The argument that is proposed in this chapter is that retained knowledge alone may not be enough in the practice of mental health therapy, and that wisdom goes beyond retained knowledge by considering such experiences as personal instincts, intuitions, and insights. In the words of Michael Polanyi, "It is in the tacit dimension where we can begin to make sense of the place of intuition and hunches in informal education practice" (Polanyi 1974). In mental health therapy, a therapist may have a more thorough understanding of client/patient suffering when set free to trust the therapy process. Or more succinctly, "We know more than we can tell" (Polanyi 1974). This may not ring true in many of the teachings when becoming a mental health therapist, but it does point to a different perception where reality is not only captured by a set of rules, procedures, and assessments. We may need to know how our client's experiences capture reality.

This was the curiosity of Frank when trying to help George in the case study. Frank had guidelines and rules through information taken from the DSM, yet tacit knowledge most likely dating back to his early childhood eventually made him experiment with entering the gibberish-oriented world that George presented to him. It was a reality based more on experience that became intuitive and offered insight into George's world. In a sense, Frank made the choice to leave a reality filled with assessments of George's condition and enter a reality that he was drawn into through instincts, intuitions, and insight.

Another phenomenon that describes this is found in classic phenomenology where the concept of *hospitality* creates an atmosphere of meaning around Frank that opens the door to George's world. In Italian the word for this is *sympatico*. Its definition is getting along and having mutual understanding with another. Deep hospitality and an inquiry into meaning are at the heart of the phenomenological approach, especially in the philosophy of Medard Boss (Scott 2002). From a phenomenological approach, the experiential therapist learns to explore meaning by the practice of hospitality and the inquiry into the interpersonal, temporal/historical, spatial, mooded, embodied, and linguistic experiences of the client. Phenomenology makes the simple assumption that symptoms have meaning, and the meaning is to be found inseparable from the person's being-in-the-world, which has these various domains as described above (Adams 2020).

As Daniel Goleman might say, it was Frank's emotional awareness and hospitality more than his understanding of the DSM that moved his behavior in a direction not covered in his clinical psychology training (Goleman 2005; Adams 2020). It was not his IQ and the ability to retain professional knowledge but his EI grounded in wisdom that directed him to the breakthrough with George.

Once, I was asked a question pertaining to wisdom during a Pod Cast with Northwestern University graduate students, where one student wanted to know how to obtain wisdom during the course of becoming a mental health counselor? My answer was, "Why do you believe obtaining wisdom starts with your professional education?" As we saw in the case of Frank, tacit knowledge can be transferable at any time. It is hard to know whether Frank's breakthrough with George was achieved through the retained knowledge in getting his degree or did it date back to his childhood where a disability made him more hospitable and gave him the wisdom to change his approach in understanding George? I told the student that at some point in his career, he may decide to go beyond his retained knowledge and use the wisdom found in former life experiences for the sake of accuracy when helping clients.

The psychologist, Carl Rogers, sheds light on the difference between knowledge and wisdom when describing the value of empathy in mental health therapy. Rogers might say, "What happens when a therapist practices empathy in therapy?" There may be statements made by the client that empathically take therapist and client in a totally different direction than what was found in a predetermined diagnosis. Rogers would say that "therapy is diagnosis" (Rogers 2015). In other words, through empathy a therapist may discover numerous shifts where the diagnosis changes and meaningful therapy may have to go in a different direction. This leads to the sometimes-asked question whether empathy finds its essence in knowledge or wisdom. Maybe a bit of both, but to undervalue the power of empathy in therapy and the wisdom it creates is to stay glued to retained knowledge that accepts reality based on the limitations of the statistical probability of the DSM.

James T. Hansen in his book, *Meaning Making and Mental Health Culture*, describes the importance of making meaning from the dialogue between client and therapist (Hansen 2018). He vividly describes how the contemporary mental health culture continues to abandon the meaning-making that emerges from serious dialogue between client and therapist, in favor of more empirical evidence set forth in the statistics-driven DSM 5. Can it be that meaning-making between client and therapist holds more validity and reliability in real-life experiences than reliance on a set of labels and a cluster of symptoms that are statistically valid and reliable but not necessarily experientially accurate? It may be a combination of the personal knowledge and experiences of the therapist found in dialogue, with the traumatic and dramatic experiences of the client, where valued meaning is found, where wisdom becomes more useful than knowledge.

"Wisdom is not a product of schooling but of the lifelong attempt to acquire it" (Einstein and Sabah 2017). The field of mental health therapy remains filled with professionals with valid and reliable acquired wisdom. Not only from their professional training but also from their unique life experiences. Again, it is important to note that acquiring wisdom does not necessarily begin with the practice of mental health therapy and being trained as a mental health therapist does not assure therapists have any guarantee of effectiveness. Knowing something and knowing your way around something are two different phenomena.

The larger problem may not lie in one's ability to use their wisdom but in whether they are given an opportunity to use it. More and more the field of mental health seems obsessed with institutional accountability which appears more valued than a therapist's acquired ability. Did you fill out your progress notes effectively? Did you make a diagnosis that is acceptable by your insurance company? Were you able to help your patient within fourteen visits allotted by your managed care plan? Did you follow the guidelines of any given disorder from the DSM 5 to assure its efficacy? Have you stayed focused on the treatment plan agreed upon in the case management meeting? There becomes much to think about in the practice of therapy in contemporary mental health, most of which is driven by controlling the process of doing therapy.

In contrast, our survival on this planet since the Paleolithic era has relied on the wisdom of certain individuals who had the personal knowledge and experience to keep us safe and help us grow. Their strength was not obtained through accountability but through ability. Obviously in a more complicated, civilized world, accountability is used in therapy to create structure and standardization, hopefully with the same goal of keeping us safe and helping us grow—at least that is the belief of more procedure-oriented therapists. The great scientist Albert Einstein said it best: "The intuitive mind is a sacred gift and the rational mind is a faithful servant. We have created a society that honors the servant and has forgotten the gift" (Einstein and Sample 1976). The same can be applied to mental health therapy, in my opinion.

Retained knowledge and obtained wisdom should not be at odds with each other. We in the mental health profession should not forget our gifts. The purpose of retained knowledge in therapy should be in service of our gifts. Wisdom is a gift we acquire through experiencing success and mistakes.

Unlike, in physical medicine where there are standard procedures for diagnosing and treatment. In mental health therapy, there are only guesses from the DSM, except for those disorders that are more pharmaceutically treated such as schizophrenia. I realize by using the word "guess" diminishes the aura surrounding the complexities described in a medical model-oriented DSM 5, so if you rather enhance its prominence one can call them "statistical guesses." Nevertheless, they are guesses, just the same. In that regard, using our personal knowledge and experience in therapy are also grounded in guesses. However, they are guesses found in the interaction between client and therapist that manifests themselves through the gift of wisdom.

More importantly, these guesses based on personal knowledge and experience have a different purpose than guesses from a calculated medical model. They are *not* statements regarding how one is labeled within the lexicon of mental health. Wisdom even though it is embedded in guesses is not to empirically determine what the client/patient "has" through a diagnostic label but to give meaning and purpose to what they "are going through" within the stories they tell and the suffering they present. In those moments in therapy, insight makes guesses come alive by giving new direction to the pathway taken by client and therapist. And, there is a subtle acceptance in such wisdom that speaks to each present moment in therapy, where both client and therapist can say, "We are in this together whether the guesses are correct or not."

NOTE

1. The statement, "It should make obtained wisdom as important as retained knowledge." This statement, I believe is one of the more ironic phenomena in medical model mental health therapy. It appears that knowledge has overtaken wisdom as our "go-to" understanding of mental disorders. However, Albert Einstein may have said it best: "I think 99 times and find nothing. I stop thinking, swim in silence, and the truth comes to me." Albert Einstein. 2013. *The Ultimate Quotable Einstein*. Princeton, NJ: Princeton University Press.

Chapter 5

Momentum versus Procedures

"When you're that successful, things have a momentum, and at a certain point you can't really tell whether you have created the momentum or it's creating you?" (Cripps 2017). This quote by Annie Lennox, the famous musician, sets the tone for the following discussion about mental health therapy, and the difference between momentum and procedures. Momentum guides the distinct sequences of events in experiential therapy, while procedures do the same for medical model therapy. Momentum is one of the untold experiences that can be monitored in therapeutic practice. Without momentum it is difficult for clients and therapist to know where they stand in the therapy process. (An exception may be techniques that ask clients to rate their progress from one to ten or similar assessments in postmodern thinking.) Yet, experiencing momentum within therapy may take a willingness to accept its importance. In a medical model, professionals rely on standardized procedures to create structure but not all experiences can be captured by this model. There may be subtle exchanges in therapy that are lost within the medical model's procedural demands.

So, what is it about momentum that makes this a phenomenon of value within the therapeutic experience? First, momentum is a force where we are connected to the world around us in an intimate way, and momentum judges the dynamics and intensity of that connection. With negative momentum in therapy, we are connected in a less intimate way, while the opposite becomes true with positive momentum. Second, we as therapists may need to create momentum in ourselves when emotionally involved in the negative experiences of our clients. One example in experiential therapy is the importance of establishing a therapeutic alliance, which tends to increase positive momentum between therapist and client. When the flow of momentum is rapidly moving in therapy, it is hard to differentiate what is driving a client toward health: the client, the therapist, or the momentum between them. In comparison, the medical model has standardized procedures that may practice numerous starts and stops when moving from one procedural phase to another, with little understanding of the importance of momentum in mental health therapy.

In experiential therapy, the therapist may choose to focus on momentum from the beginning to the very end. A commonsense reason is to change a client's negative momentum into something positive and in doing this change the direction of therapy. A client's mental health problems do not only have to be viewed through the context of symptoms, they also encompass negative momentum, where the attitude and mood surrounding the client is dynamically flowing in a negative direction. Part of forming a therapeutic alliance is to change the flow of client momentum from negative to positive. In a medical model, it becomes difficult to create momentum based on the standardized nature of procedures. Standardized procedures have the positive effect of creating more consistent therapeutic methods but do not account for the power of momentum, and in some cases, they can dissolve it.

Much of the differences are found in the thinking behind both models. Medical model therapy has copied methods from natural science where information is gathered, a hypothesis is made, a treatment plan is devised, and an execution of the plan will be evaluated for its effectiveness (Deacon 2013). In medical model therapy, these standardized procedures make patients and their experiences conform to predetermined methods, and not the other way around. The end result of this thinking is that patients will need to conform to the questions asked in the beginning moments of therapy. Their painful experiences will have to fit into some category in the DSM 5. When beginning therapy, they may have to answer another round of questions for a patient's background check before progress notes and other procedures are required by the therapist. If in the treatment plan a certain set of techniques are used, they again have to conform to the procedures, indicative of each form of treatment. During therapy they may have to conform to the judgments, analysis, and advice given by the therapist to effectively meet the goals of treatment (Farre 2017). All these procedures are commonly followed in a medical model form of mental health therapy. The more questions asked, diagnoses granted, progress notes taken, and therapy goals met, one assumes the more effective the therapy.

Experientially oriented therapists may or may not have to confront the same set of procedures depending on the location and purpose of the therapy setting. In review of the chapters in this book such themes as collaboration, wisdom, neuroscience, intuition, attunement, insight, dialogue, and experiential patterns are the foundation of an experiential therapist. Within this collection, a most important additional consideration is momentum. Included in the thinking of mental health therapists, regarding causes of mental disorders, a lack of momentum should be added to genetics, early childhood attachments, trauma, and neurological disruption of neuropathways. Experience has demonstrated that regardless of the diagnosis of genetics, lack of early childhood attachments, traumas, neurological disruption, and so on, clients/patients discover over time, if these painful experiences are not treated effectively, the intensity found in negative momentum quickly becomes an issue (Haffner 1985).

If you take a small snowball and begin rolling down a hill, at first, you will have to push it; but the bigger the snowball becomes, the more it is inclined to roll on its own momentum. Such are the experiences of those with disabling mental disorders. With the accumulation of pain over time, momentum may eventually classify their negative experiences as having a bona fide disorder. Furthermore, trauma, pain, or suffering that may take clients hours or days to resolve in the beginning, over time, negative momentum may now take clients weeks, months, or years to resolve. From an experiential perspective, negative momentum is a major reason that clients become overwhelmed with their negative experiences when they are not effectively being treated early enough, or not being treated at all. Negative momentum may be one reason responsible for the steady upsurge in untreated people for mental and physical suffering (Saxena 2019).

A therapist was working with a client who fell into a deep, negative depression. After dialogue between the therapist and client went on for a number of sessions, the client said, "I need to do something, but I am afraid that I won't do the right thing." The therapist softly remarked, "Well, do the wrong thing, but do something." The rationale for the therapist's remark was if the client did the wrong thing, then the client could try something else if it did not work. Knowing what the right thing to do was not the point of the therapist's comment. The therapist was trying restart the client's momentum. Lack of momentum toward confronting one's hurt and pain can add to the pain, or it may turn out to be the pain. This example was of a therapist trying to create positive momentum with a client knowing negative momentum had evolved into a dangerous and hurtful place in the client's life.

If one accepts the belief that negative momentum is a major concern when clients find themselves sinking into mental health problems, then gaining positive momentum becomes a valuable consideration in mental health therapy. Neurologically during a severe trauma, a person experiences neurological shock to the point of numbness and buried emotions (Siegel 2016). If a climate of safety is not emotionally established, that experience may gain negative momentum until later when an accumulative shock surfaces, causing flashbacks, dissociation, and possibly suicide ideation. The medical model labels this experience as PTSD, but experientially and neurologically, it may be negative momentum regarding unaddressed shock that becomes of equal importance as the initial shock.

ELEMENTS OF MOMENTUM

Confidence

It makes sense that in the therapy process, a level of confidence is a major element for clients to gain momentum. In a medical model, the constant emphasis on mental disorders seems less effective for momentum to happen. Metaphorically, I have emphasized with clients that it is not the "crash" as the major focus in therapy but the "bounce" they get out of it. "At some time or other we all crash. Let us use the crash as a reason to bounce back with resilience, grit and courage" (Ladd 2019). Looking for anything where a client shows some level of confidence seems an effective starting point for positive momentum. A dialogue surrounding a client's perceived competence can intrinsically motivate a client for future bouts with his or her disorder. Momentum starts as a conscious process but subsequently becomes a major facilitator of nonconscious automatic execution of human behavior and performance (Hubbard 2015).

Empowerment

Helping clients with their level of confidence at the beginning of therapy pays dividends in the dialogue later on in therapy. The therapeutic alliance important in any mental health therapy is partially based on momentum. The confidence that grows out a successful dialogue in the therapy process begins with the building of trust between client and therapist, but it is momentum that helps it move along at its own pace. In a medical model the pace is set by the guidelines and rules connected to medically oriented process. Structurally, there is little room for confidence and empowerment in therapy that moves along at a pace structured by procedures. The structured transitions from diagnosis, treatment plan, to technique practice can disrupt the momentum found when client and therapist are moving effectively through therapy.

Empathy and Selfless Acts

Empathy and selfless acts by the therapist can also build momentum. Clients may come to counseling with an extraordinarily low level of perceived competence. By the counselor practicing empathy and expressing acts of positive regard, momentum begins to grow in the client (Ladd 2018). Some clients enter therapy with negative momentum. They may be so hard on themselves that it takes establishing a meaningful dialogue to turn momentum around and go in a more positive direction. A medical model rarely addresses this issue. They focus on the disorder, not the negative momentum it is causing. Stopping negative momentum and begin building positive momentum before any serious intervention takes place is not one of the goals of medical model mental health therapy.

Intrinsic Motivation

Another aspect of momentum is found in the importance of intrinsic motivation in therapy (Hunt et al. 2013). I have believed for some years that clients want to psychologically heal, but their intrinsic motivation has yet to be discovered by themselves or by the therapist, or both (Ladd 2019). Momentum helps in finding the motivation inside. It becomes an issue of identity, where positive momentum clears the way for what clients believe about themselves. Momentum is a fully human issue, and it is stimulated by themes such as hope, insight, intuitive decisions, and attuned communication (Ladd 2019). An experiential therapist can create momentum in clients by helping to uncover their human spirit—an entity that is found in all of us, that makes us uniquely human (Frankl 2010).[1]

Mood

Moods are our brain's way of creating momentum (Hunt 2015). Successfully completing therapy is not a random event. It has something to do with your mood and the type of emotions making up your mood. If you have a breakthrough in therapy, a positive mood will be partially responsible for your success. With a therapeutic breakthrough, one can learn to expect further breakthroughs, thus creating an emotional mood for continued breakthroughs and in this manner, moods are our brain's way of creating momentum (Forte 2017). We can only have one strong thought at a time, and if our thoughts each day remain negative, we will gain momentum in creating a negative mood. The opposite is also true. If each day we try to stay positive, our positive mood can gain momentum where the next day, momentum helps us remain positive. Because we now are in *flow* and the flow helps us as much as our mood. Again, in medical model therapy, most activities are based on reducing symptoms not on changing mood. For an experiential therapist, changing a client's mood may be as important as reducing systems. When clients are in a good mood, they tend to overcome some of their symptoms. When their good mood gains momentum and they are in flow, they tend to overcome the rest of them. That is why I have admired Viktor Frankl's emphasis on humor during therapy, for its effect on creating momentum and having a positive mood (Frankl 2014).

BENEFITS OF MOMENTUM

Identity

In a medical model, changing behavior, thoughts, and feelings encompass most of the issues covered in therapy. For a symptoms reduction, symptoms maintenance model, this makes sense for most of it is obtainable or observable from an expert's perspective. In a model such as phenomenology or trauma-informed care where meaning-making goes beyond reducing symptoms, a more holistic perspective is centered around a client's identity. Attached to identity are issues such as genetics, learned experiences, and other nature/nurture phenomena that have been under the microscope of research findings for many years. Could one more consideration be made for momentum?

Could it be that negative momentum also enters into the picture of how one sees herself or himself? Could it be that the momentum of constantly increasing negativity in one's life has a dramatic and traumatic impact on identity? Furthermore, is it possible when seeking help from medical model mental health therapy, professionals have led some patients through diagnosis and diagnostic labels to experience an increase in negative momentum adding more negativity to a patient's identity? Conversely, is it possible for clients going through therapy to gain positive momentum that reinforces a positive identity, and possibly adds to the nature/nurture list as another predictor of identity? The connection between positive and negative momentum in mental health therapy is a consideration made by those thinkers who try to describe identity through client experiences not through diagnostic labels.

Character

What other benefits in therapy can be accounted for by clients changing negative momentum into positive momentum? In a medical model form of therapy, as with identity, such a question is not asked or addressed. In experiential thinking, negative and positive momentum has an impact on a client's character. The transition from negative to positive momentum in therapy builds character through the experience of suffering (Frankl 2009). It becomes an accomplishment that needs to be acknowledged for having the strength of character to make such a difficult transition. An experiential therapist tries to emphasize the magnitude of this accomplishment. It is an opportunity to reinforce client identity and begin drifting away from any diagnosis or diagnostic label.

Empowering clients to experience the journey from emotional darkness into the light of accomplishment becomes the response worthy of an experiential therapist. For example, "Look how far you have come. Once you were engulfed in negativity and now you have gained enough momentum to have pride in yourself. You have demonstrated the depth of your convictions." Having established character is something earned and should not be overlooked in the therapeutic process. If medical model therapist can point out the reality in having a disorder, then more experiential therapists may have a responsibility to point out the celebration of character, when clients transition from negative to positive momentum. Such thinking may come down to your ultimate goal in therapy. If the goal is to reduce patient symptoms and maintain a reduction in symptoms, the celebration of character is not a requirement. If the goal is to help clients grow and change, the phenomenon of momentum leading to changes in identity and character needs recognition and respect by an experiential therapist.

Grit

Awareness of a disorder and treatment through psychotropic drugs and psychological techniques may not be enough to stop negative momentum. Without the development of resilience or grit, success through medical model methods run the risk of client pain, at some point in the future, becoming overwhelming, especially during future crises. Medical model methods help control symptoms but may not control the "gritty" process of going from negative momentum to positive momentum. The field of mental health may require something beyond a psychological formula for success in mental health therapy. It may require a personal commitment by the client for mental and emotional toughness, to weather the suffering that is attached to psychological and emotional recovery. Outside influences such as psychotropic drugs and therapy techniques are important from the professional's commitment to therapy, but without client/patient commitment, therapy can become a struggle where both professional and client/patient are responsible for the final outcome.[2]

The concept of "learned helplessness" is not uncommon for those who study the process involved in mental health therapy (Cherry 2019). Neither the therapy professionals, nor the insurance companies, nor the clients themselves may want a passive outcome to the therapeutic process—except possibly Big Pharma. The experience of going through therapy is not only about reducing symptoms derived from mental disorders. It also offers the opportunity for changing one's identity, increasing one's character, and developing a certain level of grit to face future problems. Personally, I have always admired transition of those clients who at first thought of themselves as weak, believing in a negative identity, and when compared to others, felt shame, guilt, and other negative feelings, and by going through the ordeal of turning around negative momentum into something positive began feeling strong and comfortable with themselves.

Courage

The famous existential therapist Rollo May stated that "commitment without any doubt is the sign of a fanatic. True courage is commitment but with doubt" (May 1975). It may be the responsibility of experiential therapists to point out in therapy the importance of doubt when trying to turn around the momentum in client lives. Positive momentum is not without doubt. It is a myth that through the process of therapy everything now will be ok. Metaphorically, it is not waiting for the next shoe to drop but being prepared for when it does drop. Clients committed to the therapy process may occasionally have doubts. Instead of perceiving these experiences as gaining negative momentum, doubt is an opportunity to demonstrate the intrinsic nature connected to courage.

In experiential therapy, the ongoing dialogue reminds both parties that the direction of therapy may have changed, and the collaboration between client and therapist may result in the courage needed to change direction when experience demonstrates therapy is going in the wrong direction. One method that both client and therapist can assess whether this has happened is to discuss momentum during a therapy session. In my own experience, I have felt that positive momentum was alive and well in my relationship with clients, only to become aware that momentum was slowing down, placing doubt in myself or in the client. Here is where doubt allows the therapist or the client to reevaluate the direction taken. Unlike some colleagues who push the diagnosis, or push the treatment plan, or push the therapy techniques as though there was little doubt in the solutions for client/patient problems, in phenomenological thinking doubt is acknowledged as a part of human experience (May 2003). In a medical model, it becomes more difficult to have the flexibility of changing the treatment plan or the diagnosis—even though at times this does happen. In all fairness to these colleagues, I am not sure they are entirely responsible for a mental health system that requires order and efficiency at the expense of flexibility and doubt. The more a therapist or client face and work through doubt, the stronger the momentum can be in the therapy process.

CASE STUDY

Derek had just got out of prison for a combination of addiction and breaking the law that accompanied his habit. Before prison, he had been to drug and alcohol counseling, twelve-step programs, and mental health therapy. During that time, the one positive experience that seemed to have an impact on him was meeting someone with similar experiences, but had not committed any crimes, and was waiting for him after his prison release. Through his own reflections, he knew that all the labels he had accumulated from mental health, drug and alcohol, and incarceration weighed heavy on his mind—along with the perceptions of his probation officer. The basic plan was to reenter mental health therapy, drug and alcohol counseling, and to limit his association with anyone that was still using drugs. All of this was slowing down his personal plans for recovery, where freedom and a healthy relationship with his girlfriend seemed to be in jeopardy.

He came to Michael, a more experiential therapist, on the advice of a friend who had a positive experience with him and thought that he may be able to do the same for Dereck. The first meeting between Michael and Derek was not what he expected. Dereck gave Michael a history of his drug use, incarceration, and relationship with his girlfriend, and the pressures put on him by the courts and his probation officer who demanded he seek help for his addiction. Dereck seemed angry, confused and feared that his anger would bring him back to his old ways.

Michael looked at Dereck and said that he had some positive news for him. First, he asked him, "What do you think about when you are angry?" Dereck replied that he was now free and the advice from his probation officer and the courts wanted him to now go back and repeat all of the same remedies that did not work numerous times before. Michael replied, "So, those remedies did not work or is it that, as you pointed out, you are in a different frame of mind as a reason they did not work? I am asking that question because you seem different to me. Not like someone who is resisting help, or why would you be here?" Dereck replied, "That is exactly why I am here. My anger is over probation and the courts not trusting in how much work I have put into myself, and how I have changed."

"So, we are really talking about not losing your momentum in appreciating your freedom, being with a person you love, and accepting the changes in your way of seeing yourself." Dereck said, "Yes that is exactly it." Michael said, "I personally can see your dilemma; on the one hand, you feel that you have gained momentum by working on yourself, and angry about anything that would take that away. On the other hand, you are saying how scared you feel about going down the path of negative momentum that caused you to use drugs in the first place." After that brief exchange of dialogue Michael and Dereck had an understanding. There was no mention of his addiction, incarceration, criminal activity, or lack of motivation regarding past attempts to face his life. The dialogue had shifted to how would he maintain positive momentum and not fall back into the negative momentum of the past.

From that point on, they discussed what were the most reasonable possibilities in order to keep his positive momentum. He realized that if he did not obey the mandates from the court and probation officer, his anger would probably throw him back into the negative momentum from the past. He also realized that he had become a multidimensional person, who could separate his obligations to authorities combined with his love of freedom and his girlfriend. In the end, he made arrangements, on his own, to take care of the therapy obligation by having the authorities agree to seeing Michael as his means of recovery. He also applied and got a job that appeared to dramatically increase his momentum. The end result was that Dereck found a way to separate what he wanted to do from what he needed to do. At the end of therapy, Dereck left with a confident smile on his face, and thanked Michael for not judging him, and appreciating all the momentum he had gained before they met. Michael's reply was simply, "It was obvious to me that your anger was not that of a victim but of a survivor. Once you understood that, we seemed to take one session at a time to find possibilities that would keep the momentum going in your life."

DISCUSSION

The reality is that momentum becomes more of a process than a procedure or a technique that places its value out of the realm of typical medical model mental health therapy. The experiential therapist being grounded in experience, phenomena, and process places a higher value on the experience of momentum. One of the goals of an experiential therapist is to help direct negative momentum into positive momentum. Sometimes this changes the language used during therapy. In the case study, Michael did not focus on addiction, criminality, or incarceration. He perceived a person who through much of his life was building momentum through negative experiences that affected his identity, character, grit, and courage. When Dereck decided to change his life, he was intentionally talking about his identity, character, grit, and courage, though he did not know this until the dialogue with Michael put names to these experiences.

Most of his association with mental health and drug and alcohol professionals focused on the content of his behavior not on its process. That was their professional training and that was their responsibility. However, when Michael left prison, his thinking was based more on the future than on the past. His focus was on changing his identity, building character as much for himself as for his girlfriend. Proving to himself that he had a level of grit to now work through addiction and prove to himself that he had the courage to pull off his immediate goals.

In phenomenological thought, Edmund Husserl would state, "To say that thought is 'intentional' is to say that it is of the nature of thought to be directed toward or about something outside of one's self" (Husserl 2014). The intentionality of Dereck was better suited for the experiential therapy that Michael offered him. This is not to say that focusing on past behavior and feelings does not hold value. Just ask any medical model mental health therapist and they will tell you that it is highly valued, and also highly comparable to others in similar situations based on an accumulation of statistical probability through the DSM. For a phenomenological or trauma-informed care thinker, focusing on the future has as much legitimacy as focusing on the past. Experiential therapists, for the most part, are in the business of creating possibilities that will help change a client's past and develop growth and change for a client's future. Such a phenomenon as momentum enters the category of other more experiential themes such as empathy, intuition, insight, identity, courage, character, and grit. These are not symptoms reduction themes but themes based on growth and change.

Not all of a client's reality is based on what professionals can see or observe. Only those that fall under the scrutiny of statistical evaluation or experimental research seem to hold value in the current mental health culture. This should not mean that important parts of a client's reality are not valued unless they are measurable. It may mean that unmeasurable phenomena can hold equal value as measurable phenomena, when it comes to a more holistic assessment of patients/clients. Standardization of disorders should not hold a higher value than individuality of experience. There is no fine line that separates the two. In present mental health culture, there seems to be a solid thick line between them. I contend that there should be no line between medical model standardization and experiential model individuality. Metaphorically speaking, if a lumberjack and a lover look at a tree, the intentionality behind the lumberjack may see how many board feet are in the tree. A lover may look at the same tree and see the perfect spot to carve a heart in it, signifying strong feelings for their lover. This form of intentionality may be a better model than a one way fits all patient/client model of therapy. The business of mental health struggles with a more individualized personal view of reality, and banks on a more standardized view that is orderly and categorical. The question that may be asked, "Does the general public when seeking psychological help want their individual perception of reality to be the main focus, or are they looking for a more standardized version of themselves?"

NOTES

1. I have my personal list of what causes momentum and they are guts, grit, risk, and zest. The guts to face adversity, the grit to hang in there and not quit, the willingness to risk, and the zest to think with compassion. Peter Ladd. 2018. "PowerPoint Presentation," St. Lawrence University, November 30, 2018. Momentum can be as much a spiritual reality as an emotional one. Especially when the spiritual intentionality is directed at something outside of one's self.

2. "Life is like riding a bicycle. To keep balance, you must keep moving." Albert Einstein. 2013. *The Ultimate Quotable Einstein*. Princeton, NJ: Princeton University Press.

Chapter 6

Patterns versus Labels

EXPERIENTIAL PATTERNS

Experiential therapists are looking for those essential patterns that reveal some form of suffering in client's experiences, for the purpose of describing these patterns to their clients during therapy. Humans try to detect patterns in their environment all the time, because it makes learning easier. For example, if you are given driving directions in an unfamiliar city, you can try to memorize each turn. But if you see a pattern or a map, for example, turn left, then right, then left, then right, it will be easier to remember (Konovalov 2002). The same thinking is present in more practical forms of experiential therapy. Certain patterns in human experience may have common characteristics, for example, we may know when someone is being generous and when someone is not. Each of us has their unique experiences in life; however, we have in common certain phenomena or patterns that are recognizable to many different people going through these experiences.[1]

Each person may have their unique experiences with anger, but most of us recognize a pattern of anger in ourselves and in others that is vaguely familiar. The reason we recognize anger in ourselves and others is because our minds have found a way to be orderly and efficient. Many of our past experiences are perceived in "shorthand." When we have an experience in the present, we have a tendency to understand it by remembering a previous experience. We do not have to specifically remember the entire previous experience in detail but just enough of it to make the present experience recognizable in the present. In mental health therapy, we might call these vaguely familiar experiences, schematic patterns, schemata, or experiential frameworks that help us efficiently organize information as we go through life (Merleau-Ponty 2002).

Sometimes these schematic patterns may cause us personal conflict or possibly mental health problems and may hinder us from other meaningful experiences. A pattern of social anxiety disorder is a human experience that may limit our ability to socialize, or to understand the world from a more objective perspective. Though schematic patterns in our brain's memory centers tend to generalize our experiences and make them stereotypical, we continuously rely on them to understand what we are going through. Human experience is filled with recognizable patterns that may influence us on a daily basis both positively and negatively, and that has been verified through developmental learning by Piaget and others who have studied these schemata (Piaget and Endler 1972).

The experiential therapist intuitively looks for both negative and positive experiential patterns with the hope of identifying and modifying them with the client's collaborative help. Sometimes clients experience everyday patterns in living that are too narrow and inflexible. For example, a pattern of anxiety may limit what is perceived as hopeful, where clients do not notice the positive experiences before them, subsequently missing the opportunity for more certainty in their lives. These negative experiences may reinforce narrow and inflexible patterns by repeating them over and over again until these patterns become a disorder. Helping to expand these patterns of experiences or adopting new patterns of experiences is part of the mindset and belief system intrinsic in the values held by an experiential therapist.

By using an experiential approach, therapists can gain wisdom regarding the life patterns of their clients, instead of constantly referring to the DSM for knowledge regarding diagnosis and treatment. The experiential therapist goes beyond the natural scientific method in favor of an approach that asks *what clients are going through*, not by a label of what they have as a disorder. This can specifically be observed in trauma-informed care experiences. In trauma-informed care, one of the least important factors in this process is what to name the experience. The pattern remains dynamic and not frozen in time, as in labels based on statistical probability. The main intention is to help collaborate with clients about their experiences, and to develop awareness grounded in personal meaning. Unlike therapists who search for symptoms in the DSM to eventually designate a label, the experiential therapist searches for meaningful patterns in client experiences. Through dialogue and collaboration, the therapist trusts that an experiential pattern will emerge through client/therapist intuition leading to insight. Much as in the stored neurological patterns of the mind, these experiential patterns are not exact replicas of the past but close enough so personal meaning is recognizable for the client.

Using patterns to create client awareness makes pattern recognition one of the more sophisticated ways that experiential therapists develop an understanding of the human condition. The best thing we have going for us is our intelligence, especially pattern recognition, sharpened over eons of evolution (Tyson 2015). Pattern recognition according to IQ test designers is a key determinant of a person's potential to think logically, verbally, numerically, and spatially. Compared to all mental abilities, pattern recognition is said to have the highest correlation with the so-called general intelligence factor (Kurzweil 2012). The ability to spot existing or emerging patterns is one of the most, if not the most, critical skill in decision-making, though we are mostly unaware that we do it all the time (Miemis 2010). For example, a soldier may make an intuitive decision not to enter a certain dangerous location based on previous patterns that earmark danger. Therefore, pattern recognition can also help to develop wisdom.

Below is one client's description of depression. The pattern is formed by the client describing what she or he goes through when experiencing depression, while the experiential therapist tries to capture the essence of his or her experience, no matter how vague or primitive it may appear. It is a visual representation among many different ways to capture client experiences[2] (figure 6.1).

It should be noted that the "map is not the territory." For the experiential therapist, any method that can capture the meaning in client experience is more valuable than designating one method as more effective than another, and that includes using the DSM. It is not helpful to anyone in following any given method of diagnosis at the expense of having to alter a client's human experience to fit that method. (In my personal experience, when the dialogue is flowing and the meaning-making is emerging, no visual pattern seems needed to capture the essence of the pain one is going through. The client and I simply talk about it where the dialogue reveals a pattern of experience on its own. On those occasions when visualizing what a client may be feeling can help with awareness, such visual patterns appear helpful. These patterns

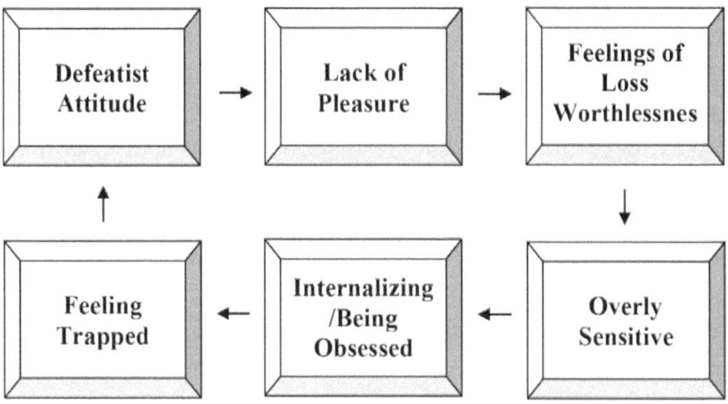

Figure 6.1 Example of a Client's Description of Depression.

are not an attempt at a diagnosis but a map or chart of the experience being discussed in therapy, especially what the client is going through.)

Let us look at this method among many others for capturing the meaning found in this client's pattern of depression. Within each phase of this pattern a collaboration is enacted between client and therapist. The therapist may share information from professional experience to inform the client of what others have reported about their experience with depression, or focus on the meaning shared by the client, and how this pattern has affected her or his meaningful experiences in the past. Through free-flowing dialogue, a pattern is recognizable. By working through the client's unique experience with depression, the client's meaning is revealed, along with discussing at each phase what can be done to find a more positive and effective approach to alleviating the pain it is causing. Depending on the intuitive decisions being made both by client and therapist during therapy, meaning may emerge simply in the dialogue itself. More importantly, in this example is a meaningful description and understanding of what the client is going through with the experience of depression revealed to both client and therapist, by talking about the patterns of experience itself.

This example demonstrates the essential value given to human experience in experiential therapy. It is treated with the highest priority, where attempts are made to clarify and rectify the damage caused by these experiential patterns. So, no matter the particular style of the experiential therapist, the ultimate goal is to capture the meaning in what clients are going through with these negative patterns. Keeping in mind, a client may have practiced over and over again a negative pattern of experience, much as neurologically the mind may have developed habitual neural pathways indicating the same negative pattern over a long period of time. What are known as mental disorders may also be perceived as neurological/experiential habits that affect both outer experiences and inner neurological pathways.

Recognizing patterns help experiential therapists predict and expect what is the next step in therapy. The process involves matching information in dialogue with clients, with information already stored in the brain of the therapist. For this to happen, neurologically, it is the parietal lobes located in the top, back portion of the brain that are responsible for spatial awareness, and for processing and analyzing sensory information (Kumagai and Akira 2010). They also play a role in focus and attention. Effective experiential therapists try to codify the way clients form painful habits in their experiences. The medical model calls these painful habits, disorders. If a therapist observes this during therapy, over time with many different clients these therapists can codify patterns that are associated with different mental health disorders. Our brain is a pattern-seeking survival machine, and habits are how it ensures that we don't have to think too hard about what to do when familiar situations arise, letting us conserve energy (Kohut 2018). However, sometimes at the detriment of the client.

Experiential therapists when asking someone "how's it going" and clients respond "great" when things are not, the face may exhibit a momentary microsecond expression of sadness. Unless you find value in recognizing such phenomena, these micro-expressions are invisible to most people. This is because these micro-expressions happen extremely fast, lasting only 1/25 to 1/50 of a second (Ekman 2007). Most anyone can be trained over time to detect these micro-expressions. Experiential therapists consciously or unconsciously are putting time and effort into these microseconds when they respond to clients through intuition, attunement, and insight, based on their added value in recognizing experiential patterns.

Patterns are a powerful part of the therapy process from an experiential perspective. They set up expectations, make connections, and inspire questions. They can be events that regularly repeat themselves in therapy. In the therapeutic relationship between client and therapist, they can create new connections, or they can emerge and help client and therapist see the larger perspective regarding traumatic experiences. Pattern recognition can lead to new discoveries, breakthrough ideas, and innovative concepts. Because the brain is wired to recognize patterns, everyone has the potential to be pattern smart. A successful experiential therapist is often involved in finding patterns where more empirical-minded therapists see nothing but a collection of symptoms (Narkman 2018).

MEDICAL MODEL LABELS

There are numerous benefits in using the DSM, and eventually arriving at a label that signifies a specific disorder. In the process of doing mental health therapy and other practices, a legitimate form of classification system was constructed. Since the beginning of the 1950s, the DSM has served as such a classification system. Along with the

International Classification of Disease (ICD-11), the DSM has been the gold standard for psychological classification of mental disorders. This standardization allows insurance companies to pay benefits for certain categories based on a patient's insurance plan. DSM standardization also benefits Big Pharma in developing drugs that can be used with different classification, for example, selective serotonin reuptake inhibitors (SSRIs) for depression or lithium for bipolar disorder. Beyond classification and payment, it also supplies managed care facilities with control over number of visits given to patients and length of these visits. Finally, some would say that it legitimizes psychiatry as a bona fide medical practice among other practices in medicine.

On the other hand, what has it accomplished for the health of patients? Some patients will actually take an inaccurate diagnosis that is covered by insurance, in order to get help. For example, a patient suffering from professional work-related exhaustion may agree to a label of depression, and be given psychotropic drugs, so she or he can receive time off from work—even though in the patient's experience with the SSRI, it may be counterproductive in treating exhaustion. Any professional therapist committed to the DSM will face such dilemmas where the patient's pain and suffering is not covered in the diagnostic book and does not capture the patient's actual experience. The compromise comes down to how much alteration to a patient's experience is a professional willing to make for the sake of being loyal to the medical model?

This leads a mental health therapist to the value placed when giving a diagnostic label. For some patients it is the practice that may save their lives from unnecessary hurt and pain. The label of bipolar disorder may explain the erratic behavior of a loved one, and ease the tensions felt by family and friends. The label of attention-deficit hyperactivity disorder (ADHD) may change the perception of teachers and parents regarding a student from a behavior problem to a problem surrounding executive functioning in the brain. In these and many other cases, the label diagnosed through the DSM may be the answer that explains to others a patient's behavior in everyday experience.

Yet, there are other side effects connected to these labels. If professionals do not take the time to understand what these experiences mean to clients, such a phenomenon as "learned helplessness" can be the end result from receiving a diagnostic label. The medical model's emphasis on symptoms reduction and symptoms maintenance leaves little room for finding the meaning behind a patient's experiences or the meaning that could be gained by patients working through their experiences to gain resilience, wisdom, growth, and change. Second, there remains the ongoing danger that by receiving a diagnostic label a patient will confuse the label with their identity. A patient may say, "Do not ask me to do anything, I am bi-polar." You cannot under any circumstances be a disorder (Ladd 2012). In medicine, patients do not say, "I am cancer" or "I am stroke." One of the benefits in phenomenology is that professionals look at client experiences and do not try to label them. In many respects, they try to externalize client experiences where they can be viewed as experiential patterns that clients are going through, not a label defining their identity. For clients to be aware of the patterns they are going through seems more advantageous than focusing attention on being labeled. As much as diagnostic labels benefit insurance companies, Big Pharma, managed care systems, and the field of psychiatry, experiential patterns benefit both client and therapist in possibilities for growth and change during the therapy process. These patterns remain dynamic and are not fixed or immovable during therapy. They do not define or describe the person but what the person is experiencing. Most importantly, they are not totally constructed by outsiders who rely on statistical probability from a professional book. They include the client as the unrecognized expert in developing these patterns.

A new study, published in *Psychiatry Research*, has concluded that psychiatric diagnoses are scientifically worthless as tools to identify discrete mental health disorders. The study, led by researchers from the University of Liverpool, involved a detailed analysis of five key chapters of the Diagnostic and Statistical Manual (DSM5) on "schizophrenia," "bipolar disorder," "depressive disorders," "anxiety disorders," and "trauma-related disorders" (Allsopp et al. 2019). Manuals such as the DSM were created to provide a common diagnostic language for mental health professionals and attempt to provide a definitive list of mental health problems, including their symptoms.

However, the following were the main findings of the research:

- Psychiatric diagnoses all use different decision-making rules.
- There is a huge amount of overlap in symptoms between diagnoses.
- Almost all diagnoses mask the role of trauma and adverse events.
- Diagnoses tell us little about the individual patient and what treatment they need (Allsopp et al. 2019).
- The authors concluded that diagnostic labeling represents "a disingenuous categorical system."

Lead researcher Dr. Kate Allsopp, University of Liverpool, said, "Although diagnostic labels create the illusion of an explanation, they are scientifically meaningless, and can create stigma and prejudice" (Allsopp et al. 2019). "I hope these findings will encourage mental health professionals to think beyond diagnoses and consider other explanations of mental distress, such as trauma and other adverse life experiences" (Allsopp et al. 2019).

In comparison, according to Tanya Peterson (2017), there are benefits to diagnostic labels such as they describe what is happening inside the patient. Labels give patients a term to explain mental illness symptoms to others. Knowing exactly what the symptoms mean can help people take effective action to treat them (Peterson 2017). They allow for efficient communication between everyone involved in someone's care, including the person herself (Peterson 2017). Diagnostic mental illness labels will likely always be used. There are students who are protected in schools by labels such as ADHD or autism spectrum disorders that shield them from being classified as behavioral problems. So, they have a function when using them for what they are—tools for protection, communication, and improvement (Allsopp et al. 2019).

CASE STUDY

Bradley was a mild-mannered man in his thirties who worked two jobs, and helped his family who were struggling to "make ends meet." On the other hand, they were not totally excepting of his lifestyle regarding his sexuality, even though they needed him. He had not come out as a gay man, and the inferences among family and friends was a constant burden to his self-esteem. Yet, his deliberate lifestyle of being dedicated to his work seemed to be a calming force in a life filled with hidden agendas and family secrets. Bradley did have a male lover who because of his secrecy took advantage of him by not telling his friends and family about his sexuality unless Bradley gave him money. This way of life was building resentful feelings in him for some time. When he became ill with hepatitis C, the pain of going through his recovery put a strain on his patience and relationships with others. The mild-mannered Bradley would flare with temper tantrums to the point that his family and his so-called boyfriend encouraged him to seek psychological help.

His first interview at the predominantly medical model mental health clinic did not improve his mood. Bradley felt the questions asked by the psychiatrist were invasive, such as "Had you felt abandonment issues as a child?" "Just how stable are your relationships?" "How do you see yourself changing?" "Can you report any emotional swings in your behavior?"—and other questions based on his present actions in front of the psychiatrist. His responses to these questions were filled with anger, even after he tried to make it clear that his bout with hepatitis C had "paid a toll" on him, physically and emotionally.

After several meetings he brought in papers for insurance purposes, in order to get reimbursed for his sessions at the clinic. At the time, the clinic's diagnosis of borderline personality disorder (BPD) 301.83 meant little to him until a relapse of hepatitis C symptoms found him early one morning in a hospital's emergency room. The nurses after reviewing his file persisted to ignore him throughout the day. Near the days end, he called family members in a rage that it was impossible to get treatment and that he was going to a specialist for further help. Family members proceeded to call the clinic and ask for guidance. They explained the symptoms of BPD and from that moment on Bradley was viewed as a disturbed person, even though he continued to bail them out financially and even though his boyfriend continued to blackmail him.

A wise colleague at work encouraged him to seek therapy where he could actually tell his story and explain his circumstances. A name was given to him, and Bradley made an appointment to see Dorian the next week. Cautiously, he entered Dorian's office and after a few gestures of saying hello to each other, Bradley went into a tirade about his family, friends, the mental health clinic, and his designated label of BPD. After a pause in Bradley's diatribe, Dorian said, "It sounds like you need to vent, so why don't you keep going." After a straight half hour of venting Bradley took a breath and asked Dorian what he thought. Dorian stated that his story points to someone who has suffered excruciating pain through recovering from hepatitis C, and he was looking for some moral support from professionals, lovers, and relatives, and he walked away with a disorder that branded him as someone who irrationally may cry for help, not because he needed it but because the judgment made was that it pertained to his disorder.

Bradley said, "That is exactly what happened to me. I was not looking for a mental health diagnosis. Nor did I count on all those I have supported over the years believing that I had a personality disorder, especially when I remain the stable influence in their lives. It is true that I have been seeking approval from my family based on my sexuality, and it is true that by not openly coming out, it has allowed my lover to blackmail me to support him." Dorian added that it sounds like his explosive behavior was in response to feeling betrayed by all involved. "Yes, that is it. I did feel betrayed. When I was in need where was everybody? I need support not a diagnostic label."

Dorian said that he would write to the mental health clinic with his permission and get his file expunged from the BPD label. "Meanwhile, why not the two of us go through some of your life experiences and look for a pattern that explains what was meaningful for you in relationship to your family, lover, and friends." Eventually a pattern emerged that described Bradley's conscious and unconscious motivation for helping so many people. Consciously, a pattern of generosity emerged where it felt meaningful to give so much to others. But right below the surface was an unconscious pattern of guilt that drove him to seek acceptance both interpersonally and sexually. The pattern of guilt emerged something like this:

> Feeling wrong—*Leading to*—Blame—*Leading to*—Shame—*Leading to*—Need for acceptance

In the following sessions, Dorian and Bradley worked through the experience of doing something wrong by coming to the conclusion that there is nothing to feel wrong about when being generous. With the experience of blame, it was a judgment he was putting on himself, and that a more appropriate feeling was to feel sad that others struggled with understanding his behavior. As far as shame was concerned, he made the decision to come out and be proud of his sexuality. Finally, he realized that it was important to accept himself rather than look to others for acceptance. He wanted their acceptance but did not need it.

When meaning was added to his experience nowhere could the diagnosis of BPD be found. That does not mean that BPD cannot be discovered by the use of the DSM5. What it may mean to experientially oriented therapists is that client life experiences may point to a disorder such as BPD or they may not. Judging patients by a cluster of symptoms and deeming them with a label does not always tell the story until client/patients become involved in the final outcome.

DISCUSSION

In a more commonsense language, if a person walked into a supermarket looking for a can of peas and there were no labels on the cans, a conflict would ensue. If the person purchased a can of peas and when arriving at home the can was filled with carrots, a conflict would ensue. The argument over whether labels in the mental health profession are important appears to be the wrong argument. In a medical model form of therapy, diagnostic labels stand for patient representations of the disorder, or disorders identifying their behavior. If the labels are accurate the mental health industry performs many tasks from insurance reimbursement to developing therapeutic treatment plans in an organized and efficient manner. The issue more accurately should be, "How do professionals ensure accuracy?" In answering this question, in an experience-oriented profession, it only seems logical for mental health therapy to consider human experience as one measure to gain accuracy. Experiential therapy whether it is oriented through phenomenology or trauma-informed care is dedicated to that consideration. Finding patterns of experience may keep in check diagnosing and giving a label where medical model labeling has a tendency to flatten human complexity for the sake of diagnosis, which shows a certain indifference to the humanistic, holistic, nuanced perspective of the client (Ladd 2009).

Experiential patterns may not be the diagnostic component that can compete with diagnostic labels when considering the business of mental health, but they can be a component that is helpful for the client. By following the collaborative dialogue between client and therapist more intuitive, insightful patterns can emerge giving clients a more dynamic form of diagnosis without the burden of supplying a label. It becomes emerging patterns themselves that help clarify what clients are going through. It allows human experience to be the focal point of therapy and not a label that, on occasions, becomes confused with patient identity. For the experiential therapist, diagnosis is more a verb than a noun. It pinpoints what someone is going through not what someone identifies with as a person. One can see this in trauma-informed care practice.

Practically speaking there are essential elements of both a medical model label and a phenomenological/experiential pattern that can be combined as benefits for client/patients. Such a combination could result in a more accurate and cost-effective cultural shift that takes into account both medical model and experiential model beliefs and behaviors. Such a shift would not only benefit the business of mental health but also benefit a more well-rounded service for the client. Granted, cultural shifts are more ominous and difficult than procedural shifts, but without the question being addressed, nothing of major significance has the opportunity to change. Carl Jung, the famous psychiatrist, stated that diagnoses should be held off until the end of therapy (Ekstrom 1988). If that were the case, diagnostic labels and experiential patterns could be combined for a more effective representation concerning an accurate diagnosis for the mental health industry.

NOTES

1. The brain is structured to be efficient and because of this, understanding neurologically and experientially *precisely* what is taking place in experience is not a valid assumption or a neurological reality. The stereotypical patterns in the brain capture the general essence of an experience not the specific drama. Therefore, experiential patterns may be more valid even though they are not statistically precise. Peter Ladd. 2018. *The Talk Therapy Revolution: Neuroscience, Phenomenology and Mental Health*. Lanham, MD: Lexington Books.

2. The experiential pattern in this chapter is based on my personal method for capturing the essential structure of any phenomena—other experiential thinkers have their unique methods of expressing these patterns. The patterns were developed by asking a wide-ranging number of clients about their experiences, and then reducing them to an essential structure. In the example described in figure 6.1, the result is not depression but a primitive map of what the client is going through. Yet, its essential structure is close enough to give meaning to future possibilities for both the client and counselor. Peter Ladd. 2013. "Knowledge vs. Wisdom in DSM Diagnosis: A Person-Centered Perspective," Article 6 VISTA, (April): Washington, DC: American Counseling Association (April 2013).

Chapter 7

Dialogue versus Discussion

In this chapter, a bio/psycho/social model of therapy will be used to show the difference between dialogue and discussion, and between a more humanistic medical model and an experiential model. In a bio/psycho/social model different types of discussions take place. Most surround distinctive portions of the therapy process where advice, questions, judgments, analysis, and encouragement are shared with patients. In the beginning of therapy, questions may be asked during the intake process. Judgments may be shared after making a diagnosis. Analysis may be given when exploring therapy techniques. Advice may be discussed during sessions at the end of therapy. Encouragement may take place when patient's run into roadblocks while accomplishing therapy goals. All of these examples show the thinking behind discussing mental health from an expert perspective. Medical model therapy uses many forms of directions to accomplish goals and plans. The type of directions used is based on a therapeutic expert trying to reduce symptoms and avoid symptoms returning.

The experiential therapist will also use these common forms of discussion in establishing issues such as a therapeutic alliance, taking in logistical information, or asking questions about one's personal environment. However, beyond everyday discussions are the invaluable free-flowing dialogues that are at the heart of phenomenological and trauma-informed care therapy. While dialogue is often confused with other forms of discourse, it belongs in a distinctive category of its own. Unlike debate, it does not involve arguing for a point of view, defending a set of assumptions, or critiquing the positions of others. Unlike negotiation or consensus-building, it is not a method of reaching an agreement or arriving at decisions. And unlike discussion, it can only emerge when participants trust and respect each other, suspend their judgments, and listen deeply to all points of view. The purpose is not so much to solve a problem or resolve an issue as to explore the most promising avenues for action (London 2018). When using dialogue in experiential therapy the direction may change many times based on the meaning that flows within the dialogue. Any discussion regarding techniques, diagnosis, and treatment plans are used only in how they fit into the ongoing dialogue between client and therapist. Most of these discussions are not at the heart of experiential therapy but are adjunct conversations based on the needs of the client—leading up to or during actual therapy.

To make a comparison, here are both communication models with the hope of perceiving the difference between them. First, here is an example of dialogue found in experiential therapy. "You said your uncle was always very fond of you, and that gave you a creepy feeling. Let us look at what creepy means in your experience with your uncle." The experiential therapist creates dialogue around the experience of being around a creepy uncle. Dialogue helps the therapist become a collaborator in the client's experience with the hope of understanding the meaning of "creepy" for the client. If the dialogue becomes meaningful and the client wants to talk about the uncle, the therapist listens until meaning is formed in his or her intuitive mind. Back and forth the dialogue might proceed with meaning emanating from the story, creating possibilities for further dialogue between the two. Or, the dialogue drifts away from the uncle and moves in a different direction to a different issue. There are open-ended opportunities for the client and the therapist to shift the dialogue to other experiences if the creepy uncle story turns out to lack meaning. Dialogue is grounded in an element of trust in the thinking and feeling of each party, and what holds meaning during their interchange within a free-flowing conversation.

For a comparison, let us contrast the experiential example with discussions held from a bio/psycho/social medical model: "You said your uncle was always very fond of you and that gave you a creepy feeling. Let us try to figure out where your thoughts are taking you. I would like to help you by using CBT to clear up your vague and disturbing thoughts about your uncle." In this example, a bio/psycho/social model form of therapy, the therapist and client discuss the direction taken toward CBT techniques included in the treatment plan. The experiential model is free-flowing. The medical model is predetermined.

Discussion in a medical model helps the therapist become an expert even when practicing empathy. For the most part, there is an intentional direction given to the client when being involved in medical model discussions. An element of control is involved in forming a conversation with clients during therapy. There are goals through an agreed-upon bio/psycho/social medical model treatment plan. In this model, it does not mean that therapists show little empathy, or they do not practice positive regard, or they lack compassion. The difference is the procedures in this model structure the discussions around the diagnosis and treatment plan. Yet, the delivery shows a more humanistic approach to a strictly executed medical model.

DISCUSSION AND THE MEDICAL MODEL

From the beginning of a bio/psycho/social medical model most discussions include numerous professional questions. In the opening interview, standardized questions are the usual practice given to most patients entering this more structured form of mental health therapy. The questions continue in forming a diagnosis ranging from "how do you feel?" to "have you ever had symptoms like this before?" The discussion continues when meeting a therapist who may have their own set of questions. In a more bio/psycho/social model, empathy and positive regard are important to the discussion making the patient feel comfortable and safe. In discussions with the patient, periodically therapists will ask questions such as: "Have you taken your meds?" "Have you practiced your homework assignment," and similar examples having to do with accomplishing tasks. All of these questions are appropriate within a model that has specific goals. Questions are meant to keep the treatment plan on track and the discussion useful. Without using numerous questions, discussions within a medical model may bog down, or the predetermined goals may go off track (Jensen 2006).

In a medical model, questions are not the only form of discussion. As trained experts, it is not uncommon for therapists to analyze specific situations and give advice. It becomes a part of the natural science methodology to problem-solve a patient's mental health issues, and to give direction through advice to next steps in patient recovery (Novak 2015). A patient may be confused when discussing some of their traumatic problems. The therapist may analyze this behavior and give advice by saying, "It may be important to stay away from your creepy uncle." Such advice is expected by patients who turn to experts to have a clearer perspective and give direction through advice.

Along with asking questions, analyzing situations and giving patients advice are what may be the cornerstone of discussions around medical model patients. In order to control mental health therapy from a medical model, whether it is a psychiatrist, psychologist, mental health therapist, or clinical social worker, the primary responsibility is to make judgments that benefit patients. Making judgments in a medical model dramatically changes the tone of any discussion during therapy. It puts the patient in the position of compliant member of the discussion. It changes from a free-flowing form of discussion to a therapist directing the exchange. The patient is put in the position of discussing answers to the judgments made by therapists as experts. For example, "When trying to get yourself out of your depression, it is important to take your meds and practice your homework." In this example, the discussion becomes more of a directive than a dialogue of ideas.

Even when medical model therapists practice more humanistic skills such as empathy and positive regard, there remains staying in an expert role where, for example, "I know it is painful for now, but this technique will eventually help you deal with your pain." Such a discussion from an expert model seems compassionate but is still making a judgment. In many respects, it puts the responsibility for recovery in the expert's hands, rather than the patient's hands. In mental health therapy, we are responsible "to" patients, but it is challenging when therapists become responsible "for" them, a common peril attached to a bio/psycho/social medical model. It is a model that shows compassion and empathy but still requires a higher level of professional control in the discussions between patient and therapist.

DIALOGUE AND THE EXPERIENTIAL MODEL

Much of the thinking regarding dialogue is common knowledge in the human science approaches to psychotherapy. It goes back to Freud but is found across the various psychodynamic, Jungian, and humanistic traditions. The most compatible example may be Robert Hobson's classic book developing a "conversational mode" for therapy: *Forms of Feeling* (1985). It is a masterful discussion of the primacy of dialogue rooted in phenomenology (Adams 2020). The late physicist David Bohm developed what is widely regarded as the most useful model of dialogue. He saw it as a method for developing what he called a "higher social intelligence." It has been my experiences that dialogue during therapy can heal the client but can also heal the therapist as well. By going beyond communication in a transcendent manner where the dialogue emphasizes a higher meaning than what is verbally communicated between client and therapist. Many breakthroughs in experiential therapy do not necessarily come from clients solely talking about their problems. Through dialogue, amazing insights emerge to the surprise of those in dialogue where the dialogue itself takes on a life of its own (Bohm 2013).

For the experiential therapist, dialogue is a form of mindful and creative contact, where client and therapist seek to set aside fears, preconceptions, or need to be the expert giving direction to the dialogue. Client and therapist take time to hear the other's voice and to create possibilities between them. Dialogue can encompass tensions and paradoxes, and in so doing, new ideas and collective wisdom may arise. It is when we let our guard down and allow our differences and doubts to surface and interact that something authentic and original can begin to emerge (Walsh 2005).

It is often in these subtle and nuanced moments in therapy that the heart and mind can come together pointing to novel therapeutic possibilities. As a therapist, one needs to remain alert to those moments, and to move with them when they arise. The most effective process for discovering these layers of meaning is through interactive dialogue, and in therapy this can lead client and therapist to something entirely new through attunement, intuition, and insight (Ladd 2018).

In experiential therapy, dialogue encourages a stream of meaning flowing among, through, and between client and therapist. It may be something entirely new, which may not have been in any medical model treatment plan. It is something creative, where this shared meaning is the "glue or cement" that holds people and societies together (Dodd 2015). Dialogue is that conversation in which therapist and client think together in relationship to each other. Thinking together implies that you no longer take your own position as final. You relax your grip on certainty and listen to possibilities that result simply from being in relationship with another (Valtanen 2019).

Underlying Structure of Dialogue

In previous chapters the discussion turned to the importance of patterns in the practice of experiential therapy. The following is an attempt to capture the essential structure or pattern of human dialogue. The actual content of any successful dialogue is unique and signals creative moments in communication. We turn to the pattern or underlying structure only for a better understanding of the phenomenon itself. Keeping in mind that the following is only a pattern or a map of dialogue. In order to fully understand it, one must practice the real thing. These primitive series of phases cannot capture the many meaningful nuances involved in true dialogue.

In the Beginning

In the beginning of a therapeutic dialogue, there may be little deep meaning indicated when client and therapist are getting to know each other. There could be discomfort, curiosity, anxiety, and many other possibilities when both parties are focusing on the initial contact between them. Most likely those opening sessions will be more along the lines of regular discussions where both parties may ask questions, give opinions, and so on. If the therapist is closely attuned to the client, certain subject matter may come up that creates common ground between them. For example, both may like to go fishing and within what may seem as small talk, a visceral connection hopefully begins. If objective information is required by the institution, then it may be the responsibility of the therapist to make a point that therapy has not yet started until intake work is completed (Ladd 2012). Personally, I believe a therapist needs to get closure on this process with a client before sharing the pain of client experiences.

Coming Out

When actual therapy has begun, and the clients begins to share their experiences, it seems important to understand that the client is vulnerable but has decided to risk sharing themselves in a meaningful and sincere manner. It is at this point in creating dialogue, where a therapist defines her or his role in the therapy process. From a medical model what is being said by the client could be questioned, analyzed, judged, or encouraged. From an experiential perspective, it intuitively and empathically means the therapist is also going to be vulnerable and get in touch with what he or she is thinking and feeling at the moment when the client begins sharing.

Putting Your Thoughts and Emotions Aside

The next phase in creating dialogue shows the counterintuitive and sometimes paradoxical nature of having a dialogue with another person. Most of the time in discussions, we get in touch with our thoughts and feelings and then talk back to the other party based on these thoughts and feelings. If they come out with anger, we may respond with anger. If they come out with love, our feelings and thoughts might turn to love. However, when you put your thoughts and feelings to the side and get in touch with what the client is thinking and feeling, true dialogue begins. In therapy, dialogue is not a reaction to what someone else is saying but an action to connect with the client. You are making no assumptions about what the client literally says. You are open to what emerges from this interactive dialogue only in a hospitable and non-analytical manner, where the focus is on the meaning behind the dialogue itself.

Look through the Client's Perspective

Metaphorically speaking, it now becomes the process of looking through the eyes of the client. It is an attempt to enter their world and look at it through the client's lens and see the world that brought them to therapy. Sometimes this is difficult to accomplish if you are struggling with your personal thoughts and emotions and are having difficulty putting them aside (Ladd and Blanchfield 2016). If both client and therapist feel safe through establishing a therapeutic alliance, the connection through dialogue is made easier. It is hard to imagine dialogue taking place in an unsafe environment. Dialogue becomes more than a discussion between two people. There is an innate human connection that Martin Buber would call the healing power of dialogue (Buber 2002).

Talk

It is at this point, in my view, where the experiential therapist becomes more sophisticated than a medical model therapist. After getting in touch with your thoughts and feelings and putting them aside, and then having looked through the client's perspective, you are now in a position to intuitively say whatever is on your mind and for the client to say whatever is on her or his mind. It is this alliance between client and therapist that makes whatever follows richer, more meaningful, and more open to change. At this point, who knows what will be said to each other. It may be the meaning behind the message that is being sent between the client and therapist that creates successful dialogue, rather than an accumulation of objective information that renders a discussion from an expert therapist viewpoint. Dialogue may imply the following: I hear you. I feel your pain, I am with you in starting this process. You can trust me. We will do this together. You are not alone. Herein lies the power of the meaning behind dialogue where intuition, attunement, and insight become possible in the healing process and a certain *hospitality* exists that encourages healing. Dialogue may be the same healing process that has allowed us to coexist for thousands of years on this planet. It is not necessarily what is said but what it means while both parties collaborate on client experiences.

Adjust Your Delivery

I have observed highly competent experiential therapists change their delivery in mid-sentence because they realized what was being said was not working. The therapist was not attuned to the client (Ladd 2018). Your ability to have a dialogue allows both parties to use a different set of skills in the free-flowing experience between client and therapist. It is where intuition, attunement, and insight take over the flow of meaningful experiences. I am still amazed that when in dialogue with clients how quickly I realize when it is not working. In some ways, when the dialogue is in flow and is humming along, it may become a shock to the unconscious mind when suddenly it is derailed by an unrelated comment of the therapist.

One final note, the above-described pattern of dialogue takes a split second to happen. When the pattern is viewed in incremental phases as described in this chapter, one realizes that "the map is not the territory." It takes practice to experience true dialogue where Martin Buber (2002) states, "There are three considerations when trying to understand dialogue; the client, the therapist and the dialogue itself." The dialogue itself helps in the healing process if allowed to flow freely between client and therapist in real time.

CASE STUDY

The following will follow a trauma-informed care model. It will emphasize the importance of safety but also the value in a free-flowing dialogue between therapist and client.

Kamia was a teenage victim of domestic violence, sexual abuse, and growing up within a climate of drugs and alcohol. She had been in and out of foster homes after being taken away from a home that was filled with neglect and a family that had scattered to different parts of the country. Presently, she was residing in her fifth group home for children and classified with oppositional defiant disorder or conduct disorder, though her behavior was more defiant and violent than sadistic or cruel. She had a history of meeting with therapists who diagnosed her with ODD but had little success in getting anywhere with her violent behavior. The dramatic behavior that shocked therapists, administrators, and professional social workers was when bullied or backed into a corner, she had a tendency to stab whoever put her in that position. Because of this, her reputation followed her wherever she landed, after being rejected by the former institution or therapist.

Her present living conditions were in a group home for girls where the other residence knew of her reputation and stayed clear of any close contact with her. The rumor was that she had stabbed five other girls, which was a well-known story that frightened these girls and also the professionals at the group home. Recently, in the community where the group home resided a trauma clinic opened in a small one-story house with a living room, bathroom, and a kitchen with appliances. In the kitchen there was bottled water in the refrigerator, snacks on the counter, and an atmosphere that was made to express comfort and not a typical clinical setting. Sometimes the home was used to interview victims of violence, rape, and abuse by professionals who would gather together to interview these victims and determine what was the appropriate direction to take in their behalf—sometimes legal, sometimes therapeutic, sometimes both. However, on Tuesdays and Thursdays the house was designated for a trauma specialist to see different clients throughout the day.

Pedro was a licensed psychologist, who had spent many years working with victims of trauma and was finding that recently his more trauma-informed care style of therapy was highly successful with teenagers, both male and female. The professionals in Kamia's group home heard about this success and scheduled an appointment to see Pedro one morning on a Tuesday. They informed him that no one had been able to control her, and that her reputation proceeded her everywhere she was placed. They basically reported that there was nothing that could be done, and they believed she would eventually end up serving time in jail.

The first meeting between them was interesting for those who have an obsession with personal dynamics. Here was a teenage female talking to a middle-aged male, and you would think they had virtually nothing in common. At the moment when they met, there was one obvious thing they did have in common. Both were checking each other out as to how this would work out. Pedro, for whatever reason, began to smile as Kamia told how him how she felt about the group home, the places she had terrorized, and specifically, him. She stated, "What in hell do you think you can do for me?" Pedro responded, "Would you like some bottled water?" This took Kamia back, sort of in shock. "Why do you ask me that?" Pedro said, "I don't know but you looked thirsty." Kamia responded, "Sure." Pedro went to the refrigerator and got two bottles of water and gave one to Kamia where they both took a moment to have a long drink from the bottles. Pedro also mentioned the snacks in the kitchen if or when she may be hungry. She shyly nodded her head.

That was the contextual extent of the first meeting beyond small talk about other girls in the home, and how she thought most of them were fools. Near the end of the session, Pedro asked, "Before you go would you like to take some snacks with you." Kamia went to the kitchen where there were placed boxes of different types of packaged snacks from cookies, crackers to sealed packages of muffins. As she walked back into the living room where they had been talking, she posed a sarcastic look on her face as though she had gotten away with something. Her jacket and pockets were stuffed with packages. She was giving Pedro a quizzical look as to what he would say about her obvious overindulgence of taking as many packages as possible. She wanted to see just exactly what he would say. Whether he would judge her for what she had done or what exactly would be his response. Pedro looked at her and laughed, "Seems like you were hungrier than I thought, but that's ok, enjoy yourself."

For a teenager who had spent most of her life defiant of authority, Pedro's mood, demeanor, and behavior were different. On the next visit, she shared her love of fashion, and how she looked forward to shopping for nice clothing. Pedro made a point to comment on her impeccable choice of clothing that she was wearing and were her jeans just old or was there a purpose for holes in them. For the first time she broke into a smile and said, "You really don't know how people dress these days." Pedro said, "I guess not why don't you tell me." Kamia began describing intricate differences in clothing and fashion in general, also continuing to tell him how little he knew. Pedro admitted it was not something he cared much about, but the way she was excited about it made him feel happy that she was happy. At the next meeting, Pedro had purchased some fashion magazines and a similar conversation took place but in a more relaxed and informal way. The professionals later asked him what he had done with Kamia. She is coming back from sessions being calm and has actually helped some of the girls with their makeup and clothing.

There was no doubt a therapeutic alliance was forming, and the visits appeared helpful to Kamia, and Pedro actually enjoyed them as well. After there was comfort between them, Pedro asked her, "If I start talking about some of the trauma you have been through, and you will not stab me, will you?" Most may believe such a bold statement would cause anger, resentment, or revenge, but Kamia smiled and said, "No I will not stab you." She then proceeded to describe the superficial stabbing she inflicted mostly on other girls, where she would break the skin but not go for any vital organs. She described exactly where to stab so no damage was done. She also described girls who would slash you with a knife, and how that was not considered high-class and did not meet the standards of a good stabbing. The rest of the session was spent in Kamia describing her unusual value system concerning what she would and would not tolerate.

Between the next Tuesday, Pedro dwelled on what she had said about stabbing, her system of values, and her obvious attempt to protect herself from others. He realized that if you took away her abhorrent behavior, she appeared a highly independent person with strong values concerning what she liked and disliked, what she respected and did not respect, and what she was willing to emotionally share if given the chance of not constantly being judged and not being feared by others. In their next meeting he began to see a different Kamia. The toughness was gone, and she was exploding with thoughts about things she wanted to do, and where she wanted to go. Here is a small example: she wanted to grow herbs and plant in a garden of turmeric, because she read about its health benefits. She started thinking, when older, about being a fashion designer. She wanted to help children who were going through similar circumstances. Pedro's response to this small sample was to find out how to grow turmeric and when to plant it, to bring books of fashion and have her educate him, and to help her get a volunteer position in giving out food at the local food pantry.

Beyond all of this was her willingness to begin talking about the traumas in her life. It was clear to her that she did not have to discuss anything she did not want to discuss. Pedro told her that sometimes keeping trauma inside creates more trauma and getting it out in the open makes it less threatening and more obvious. Many of the sessions were focused on getting out the trauma. She was even willing to try EMDR. She eventually began using it to control her anger. Pedro felt that Kamia had changed not by focusing on what had happened to her, or even on her aberrant behavior, but on what was meaningful in a life filled with trauma, violence, and pain. It was not that her valuing independence was dangerous, but the methods she used to protect herself were dangerous. It was not that she had a defiant personality, but it was her negative experiences that defined her personality. When the focus switched to what she had gone through, her behavior became clearer and made sense. Within all of the meetings between Pedro and Kamia, a free-flowing dialogue kept taking them to places that seemed unrelated to professional trauma therapy. Yet, the dialogue itself helped Kamia heal both internally and externally. As for Pedro, his responsibility was to trust the process and trust the dialogue would find a level of integration between them. He attuned to Kamia's experiences through empathy. He avoided judgments, analysis, and questions and let his intuition run freely. He allowed himself the potential for having insight, no matter how unusual it may appear to other professionals. Dialogue gave him permission to do all these things.

DISCUSSION

Dialogue and discussion are two words that can be confusing when practicing mental health therapy. How do we define the difference between dialogue and discussion when using a medical model or a more experiential model, and in this case, a trauma model? A dialogue is a conversation that takes place between two or more people. In the dialogue between Pedro and Kamia, there was a free flow of communication as they exchanged their ideas, and also responded to the thoughts and feelings of each other. In a medical model, discussion becomes different than dialogue, although in a discussion we also exchange information as the therapist talks to the client. The key difference is that most discussions are decision-based as can be seen in a medical model form of discussion. Decisions are made during intake, diagnosis, treatment plans, and acting out treatment plans. During these procedures the flow of ideas is often disrupted as professionals make an attempt to prove the validity of their diagnoses, rather than being open to the ideas of others. In a dialogue, making decisions is not the key component. In discussion, making decisions *is* the key component. A medical model uses many forms of discussion to make decisions the key component in analysis, judgments, advice, questions, and even encouragement. Discussion uses all of these to decide on a diagnosis and treatment plan. In experiential therapy, all of the above forms of discussions may be used, but the key component is the free-flowing experience one finds in dialogue.

For many professionals in the field of mental health therapy, the beginning sessions between Pedro and Kamia could be classified as small talk or icebreakers, but in trauma-informed care they were much more. The subtly and nuances of dialogue make every small gesture a part of the healing process. It is the nuances, the gestures, the glances, the moment-to-moment rhythm between Kamia and Pedro that allow the dialogue to continue in a free-flowing experience of healing. Some would say, "What about the real stuff?" "Where is the debriefing for trauma?" "Where are all those therapy skills that were learned when becoming a therapist?" They become important when Kamia and Pedro are ready to benefit from them. EMDR was eventually used when Kamia cared about Pedro enough to go along with his request for the skill. This raises the question of whether mental health therapy is a skill-based, decision-based profession? Or, is it the connection between two human beings looking for healthy possibilities in healing to change the direction of one's experience of pain and suffering?

Chapter 8

Nuances versus Symptoms

Merriam-Webster defines nuance as "a subtle difference in or shade of meaning, expression, or sound" (2019). In the field of mental health therapy, the experiential therapist defines nuances as gestures that are filled with subtle meaning that go beyond obvious communication between client and therapist. Nuances become an important phenomenon when creating a dialogue that gives meaning and direction in the therapy process and are more than nonverbal gestures. They often signify something deeper and more meaningful as signs of where therapy is heading. In comparison, a medical model form of mental health therapy is more concerned with recognizable behavior that pertains to client symptoms in exchanges between patient and therapist. A medical model therapist may observe symptoms such as a lack of pleasure, low mood, change in appetite, and so on. These are recognizable symptoms that are classified under certain disorders, in this case, depression. They are not connected to meaningful dialogue but to references in the DSM 5.

Experiential therapists may observe similar symptoms found in a pattern of depression, but they are looking for the subtle nuances that give direction while creating dialogue between client and therapist.[1] In contrasting nuances with symptoms with the above example of depression, a client displays tears when mentioning a specific incident or story. That nuance may lead the therapist to mention, "Can you put meaning to those tears, and how they relate to your experience of depression?" Or, a client may smile when describing an experience that signifies moments when depression has lifted. The therapist may ask, "What is the meaning behind that smile?" Such nuances are not a part of obvious symptoms, in this example of depression. The experiential therapist may direct the dialogue in an entirely different direction based on this nuance. The philosopher, Maurice Merleau-Ponty, wrote an article called "Cezanne's Doubt," where Paul Cezanne, the famous artist, would look at his paintings from many different angles until a specific nuance directed him to make the next stroke on the canvas (Merleau-Ponty 1992). In the field of mental health, there may be certain nuances by the client that hold a history of meaning that intuitively connects with insights found in the therapist's understanding of the problem. This helps in changing the direction of therapy. It may be why some critics call experiential therapists more artists than technicians in their ability to follow a nuance, much as Paul Cezanne followed the correct nuance that added to a stroke on the canvas. As Paul Cezanne would reiterate, "The landscape thinks itself in me and I am its consciousness" (Danchev 2013).

Experiential therapists act in a similar manner when intuition, insight, instinct, or risk captures a meaningful nuance from the client that subtly defines the direction or the essence of the client's pattern of experience.[2] These nuances do not originate as symptoms in a book such as the DSM. They are captured in "real time" and give meaning to individual stories that clients go through. Individual experiences where the nuance captures the essence of the experience, emotionally, cognitively, or behaviorally. It is not a predetermined symptom from a predetermined manual. When real dialogue is at work, the therapy session becomes a rich environment filled with nuances, looks, or gestures that direct both client and therapist into a better understanding of the reasons behind the existing problem—many times without anything being spoken or described. As Polanyi points out in chapter 4, "We know more than we can tell." Subtle nuances may signify the actual suffering that a client is going through and it may be our tacit personal knowledge found in our unconscious mind that clings to the actual meaning of suffering for the client (Scholl and Hansen 2018).

With a medical model therapist, much of what is gathered and evaluated are symptom clusters that pertain to a specific disorder found in the DSM. For example, those symptoms that statistically match with PTSD. For the experiential therapist, understanding the underlying traumatic experience of PTSD through the eyes of the afflicted person is where the focus is directed—on those experiential clues or nuances that identify the trauma in that moment in therapy. Nuances can make a difference in meaning. For example, the nuance of client discomfort observed by the therapist when talking about a family member. Such a nuance could be an opening in exploring abuse, family conflict, or anything else. Many times, nuances precede and send the signal that some underlying experience is trying to surface. These are clues filled with meaning, not behavioral or emotional symptoms that legitimize a DSM diagnosis. They may show behavior and emotion, but they signal a deeper meaning for the client. For example, the sadness that comes over a person's face when talking about the loss of a loved one.

Unfortunately, nuances become more difficult to describe in a more increasingly empirical world. I was talking with a colleague of the difficulty writing this chapter. I told him describing the symptoms of mental health therapy seemed remarkably clear, but the nuances kept escaping my thoughts and writing. He said, "Let me help you." He described being at his daughter's wedding, and during the reception afterward his daughter said to the group, "This is for my dad." She played the song from her childhood that he used when putting her to bed at night. As soon as he heard the song, he broke into tears. He said it was one of the highlights of his life. Nothing was said and everything was said. It captured the love and respect she held for him. It was a nuance that stood for a lifetime of meaning between the two of them.

In therapy, similar nuances can change the direction in therapy. I was working with a young woman who led a life of prostitution, and in therapy she understood what to say and how to say it in a very programmed way. I listened to her pattern of avoiding her emotions until she started talking about her son. She desperately was trying to regain custody. Up until this point, there was little true dialogue taking place. It was more of a discussion about her working habits. When she first started talking about her son, a sincere tone of voice formed in her communication. From that point on, the dialogue took a turn toward love, loneliness, and meaning for herself and her son's future. Even though her diagnosis was antisocial personality disorder, those symptoms dropped away when the quick, but undeniable nuance took place. It changed the entire dialogue, and it led to a positive outcome in therapy.

It seems that nuances can take the most inauthentic conversation between client and therapist where it suddenly captures the meaning behind what the conversation really means and not necessarily what was said. The combination of forming the safety of the therapeutic alliance and the capturing of meaningful nuances can change a therapy discussion into a therapy dialogue, where both parties begin looking for avenues of possibilities so healing can begin. I compare nuances to fine poetry. A poem can say in a few words and create a thousand possibilities. Nuances are subtle inflections or gestures that create in therapy a similar experience. As stated in previous chapters, momentum, dialogue, experiential patterns, collaboration, and even wisdom can emerge from meaningful nuances. It is the real-time capturing of nuances that allows experiential therapists the freedom to follow these subtle gestures wherever they may take them. In my experience, putting my trust in the hands of nuances expressed by clients has added to my belief that following nuances are more accurate than following symptoms. Client problems seem to come closer to expressed nuances than observed symptoms of clients.

It may be that the key to experiencing nuances in therapy can be credited to the experiential therapists who practice a disciplined naivete (Merleau-Ponty 2002). This is a phenomenological term for clearing your mind of assumptions, and stopping the chatter found in thinking, and letting nuances in therapy begin to emerge. Capturing nuances is not a cognitive experience. One may credit it more to mindfulness (Williams and Penman 2012), or again a discipline naivete, where you allow yourself to be open to the experience in a disciplined way.

Experiencing the nuances of clients in therapy may require acts of trust, rather than acts of control—an ongoing problem to grasp or understand in empirically oriented mental health therapy. Most of the medical model in mental health is grounded in control: control of the initial interview, control of the diagnosis, control of the treatment plan, and control of reducing symptoms. In contrast, an experiential model of mental health is grounded in trust: trust in collaboration, trust in the dialogue, trust in experiential patterns, and trust in nuances that lead client and therapist to the heart of many issues in therapy.

These phenomena may discriminate the difference between an empirical mind and a curious mind. The empirical mind of the mental health therapist is based on controlling the therapy process. It relies on statistical probability of the DSM, the efficacy of techniques, and the acknowledgment of symptoms. The experiential mind of the mental health therapist works from a more curious standpoint. A mind that is curious about forming a therapeutic alliance with each unique client, a mind that is curious about creating an effective dialogue, a curious mind that does not focus on disorders but on client experiences, and a mind that is curious about specific nuances that act as a gateway into the meaningful experiences of each unique client. This makes trust a key ingredient for a curious mind.

Curiosity in mental health therapy is a strong desire to know and learn something about the experiences of clients. Empirical knowledge in therapy is acquired by means of the senses, not through curiosity but by observation and experimentation. The curious mind of the experiential therapist is most interested in nuances that stand for something meaningful in the experiences of clients. The empirical mind of the medical model therapist treats symptoms that are statistically proven to authenticate a mental health diagnosis. Medical model mental health therapy is more controlled by science. Experiential mental health therapy is formed around an act of trust in human experiences shared in the dialogue between client and therapist, which needs to be preceded by a therapeutic alliance.

The basic attitude with the medical model therapist relies on the empirical collection of probable symptoms that can justify making a diagnosis based on some form of disorder. The experiential therapist remains curious about the negative and positive experiences that the client has gone through. There may be certain nuances that capture the curiosity of the therapist that are not obvious to the empirical mind. The curious mind of the therapist looks for these nuances and subtleties. The therapist's curious mind looks for nuances that pop up from tacit knowledge streaming from the unconscious mind. The empirical mind looks for predetermined symptoms to validate a hypothesis. A curious mind is looking for possibilities. An empirical mind is looking for probabilities.

The medical model therapist's ultimate goal is to find a diagnosis and treatment plan that reflects the most accurate form of probability from knowledge found in the DSM. This is accomplished to ultimately reduce the patient's symptoms. The ultimate goal of the experiential therapist is to work through experiences with the end result being the creation of numerous possibilities for the future. In mental health therapy, probability is about getting as close as accurate to a pathology—a typical modernist, natural scientific inquiry. Possibility is about what avenues of meaning can come out of a so-called pathology. Nuances lead to client possibilities. Symptoms lead to client probability of some type of disorder. Symptoms are based on *identifying something*. Nuances are based on *working through something*. This phenomenon can be explicitly observed, for example, in trauma-informed care, narrative therapy, and other postmodern skill applications.

In medical model mental health therapy, symptoms represent empirical observations that try to be as precise as possible through the use of statistical data, and in this way, symptoms are established as guidelines in therapy. In experiential mental health therapy, nuances represent an introduction into meaningful experiences that are not necessarily precise but comprehensive, where the whole experience is revealed, not grounded in statistical data but in meaning-based data—not to establish symptoms but to establish an accurate perspective. Experiential therapy does not want to look at pieces of a client's disorder but to see the client as a whole human being within their world of experiences. Not to label the client according to a disorder but to understand the pattern of experience that has become dangerous to the client's well-being.

CASE STUDY

In the mid-1950s, Paul Big Water entered a residential school in Ontario, Canada. These were government-sponsored facilities along with administrators from the church for the purpose of educating and assimilating indigenous children into Euro-Canadian culture. Children were rounded up from Aboriginal Reservations and taken to these schools, and Paul Big Water was one of them. In 2015, the Canadian government was making restitution for the many abuses that took place while in these schools housing Native children. Child abuse, rape, corporal punishment, and malnutrition were some of the reasons for eventually closing down the residential schools, because they were becoming a legal problem.

The ironic state of affairs for Paul Big Water was that the courts in Canada were looking to give another residential student from one of these schools' financial restitution. The residential school student had informed authorities of Paul's involvement in his experience of rape, as a young child while attending the school. Presently, Paul was not a young adolescent but a man in his late sixties who had harbored strong memories of his own experiences at the school. The courts wanted to know whether the claimant was telling the truth, and Paul's possible involvement in the climate of the school. The courts sent Paul to a medical model mental health therapist who took copious notes about his experiences at the residential school, and had him try to recall his connection with the claimant and report back to the Court whether he was also traumatized by the experience and was suffering from PTSD. This diagnosis had a severe impact on Paul to a point where he was experiencing suicide ideation. Paul's lawyer felt that the diagnosis and conclusions began to put Paul over the edge of his capabilities to deal with the entire experience.

Paul's lawyer and family became extremely concerned about his mental health. It appeared to them that being a suspect in another child's experience of rape had re-traumatized him. Over the past fifty years, he had become an upstanding member of his Reservation, and had started a highly successful marine construction company, and in a matter of weeks he felt his reputation had been destroyed, even though he experienced many of the same atrocities as his accuser. The family decided that he needed to talk, but not with a someone who only talked about his symptoms. Fortunately, a mental health counseling center did exist on his Reservation with a more holistic approach that coincided with the culture of the Native people living there.

His meeting with Peter, a middle-aged white man, was his referred to mental health therapist, and would have been a shock, if he was not told of Peter's long-standing experiences with Native people. Nevertheless, Paul was uneasy about meeting him and sheepishly walked into his office. Peter had some information about Paul that seemed to take him back when asked, "I here you are a pretty good marine contractor, and I am trying to decide whether to go with a pole dock or a crib dock. I am building a dock on this river-front property, so I wondered whether you had any ideas?" A smile covered Paul's face when he asked, "Is the river bottom mud or do you have rock?" Peter said, "It is mud." Paul replied, "I would go with a crib dock for more stability even though it might cost a bit more in materials." Peter thought to himself that Paul's smile was good sign. He was open to talking about something that had not been tarnished by the residential schools.

At the end of the session, Peter told Paul that they can talk about his situation anytime he was ready, but there was no rush. Paul later told his lawyer that Peter showed him respect, and how important that was to him. Peter saw Paul's face turn from embarrassment to respectability initially by the nuance of a smile, and that started the discussion between them. It was obvious to Peter that respect had been an important part of his life, and he appreciated someone recognizing it. Peter knew that honor and respect were highly valued on his Reservation; however, it was the moment that Paul looked at him with embarrassment that Peter intuitively, and in an instant, knew what to say. The look of embarrassment and a smile turned the conversation to marine construction, regardless of how superficial one would judge this experience. Initially what was happening in the therapy between Peter and Paul was not small talk. It was not an "icebreaker." It was a concerted effort by Peter to form a therapeutic alliance with Paul, so when ready he could pursue the trauma that was on his mind.

The dialogue followed when Paul was ready to talk about the courts, the student at the residential school, and about himself. Again, he smiled at Peter, but was a different smile based more on irony than on a personal connection. Paul, with a sarcastic look on his face, explained that here he was having worked most of his life to be a good person, and trying to put the residential school behind him, and now he was accused of victimizing someone else when he was a victim himself. He then broke down, cried, and shared his biggest humiliation would be if his grandchildren found out about all of this. He was their hero, and now he had the tone of betrayal in his voice. Peter shifted the conversation to Paul's love for his grandchildren, and a mixture of happiness and sadness covered his face. Peter said to Paul, "Whatever we accomplish here in therapy will be dedicated to their name." That struck a chord with Paul. He said that he would do his best to tell the truth as he remembered it and make his grandchildren proud.

The next session Paul described the sexual abuse, the rape, and humiliation that he endured for four years. At one point, he thought the alleged rape of a former student may have happened in the boiler room where he and some older guys did what had previously happened to them, though he could not remember ever raping anyone, and he could not remember the boy in question. All he could remember was the guilt, shame, and humiliation found in the administration of the school. He broke down and cried because he wanted to remember but could not remember. As it turned out, his accuser in his own pain and suffering realized that it was not Paul but a young administrator that looked like Paul. You would think this news would be a relief to Paul, but he was too far into his own trauma from the school that he felt sorry for the victim and believed they were both suffering the effects of abject cruelty from the residential school experiences.

Peter realized that finding out from his accuser that it was not him did little to move the specter of embarrassment and humiliation that hung over

Paul's head. For the rest of the therapy, Paul was given the chance to vent all those atrocities that he experienced during adolescence. Peter picked up in Paul a different concern, a concern that was reflected in his eyes. Finally, Peter said to Paul: I think we are at the point where you have the option to choose whether to continue as a victim or transform yourself into a survivor. It would be impossible to describe why he thought Paul was ready for that challenge, but certain nuances from Paul said he was ready. The rest of therapy was spent on how he would confront his family, grandchildren when older, and explain what it meant to survive trauma and adversity. Though Peter set the stage for Paul to reach this point in his life, it was Paul who took a stand against the cruelty of a life experience that no one should ever have to experience. Later, Paul gained respect in his community by coming out and sharing his story.

DISCUSSION

In mental health therapy, nuances seem to open the door to epiphanies—moments in therapy that change the direction of the story being told. Not all the time but for the experiential therapist, valued at the level of importance as symptoms connected to disorders. If a therapist is focusing on the experiences of certain nuances, a door may open to intuitive grasps of reality, illuminating discoveries, realizations, disclosures, or insights that change the client and therapist in some way. We see this, in the case study, when Paul had this moment of sorrow for himself and the accusing former student from the residential school. It reflected in his eyes, when Peter challenged him to make a choice between being a victim or a survivor. It was the turning point in Paul's recovery. It was an epiphany.

Wrapped up in these moments, for the experiential therapist, are any number of other phenomena that can be happening at the same time. A sense of collaboration is shared regarding the intentionality of the client. The importance of dialogue emerges. The moment gains momentum that carries the deepest sense of awareness to what is at stake. An experiential pattern is revealed replacing a mental disorder and its label. All of these phenomena happen when the door is opened through nuances. In more everyday examples, nuances are those subtle articulations that uncover the meaning in a moment when a person is touched by a poem, moved by a work of art, or becomes aware of deep human meaning in therapy. These discoveries will not happen under the umbrella of the empirical mind. They require a curious mind to unlock their secrets. In all of the above examples, it requires the curiosity of the observer to trust the process whether a poem, a work of art, or human experiences in therapy.

The medical model has uncovered information that holds importance for the therapist and patient regarding healing but so also does the experiential model in its humane treatment of client's experiences. Nuances created during experiential mental health therapy may be considered mere behavioral gestures to the empirically minded therapist. To the experiential therapist, awareness of nuances can be the turning point for potential growth and change. For example, I was celebrating the accomplishment of a friend's son in receiving a PhD in chemistry. I said to him, "You must be so proud of your son getting a PhD." He said,

> "When my son was in the second grade they were handing out awards at the end of the year. I watched as each student in the class went up to receive an award except my son. I remember the look as he turned around and stared at me, with failure written all over his face. At that moment, no matter what he did or what he accomplished, I was never wanting to see that stare again. I talked to him later, and discussed the importance of trying and not necessarily in succeeding. I am here to celebrate his 'grit' not his PhD, and he knows that."

The curious mind translates such examples into pure meaning that do not require empirical evaluation. Mental health therapy is full of these moments, if the therapist remains curious to the meaning behind a client's life experiences. These moments happen not to prove any diagnosis or to accomplish any mental health procedures. They are reflections of the intuitive mind at work. These reflections seem to appear most often when there is an established dialogue between therapist and client. To quote Martin Heidegger, "Life is not a problem to be solved but a mystery to be lived" (Heidegger 2019). It may be that nuances remain a bit of a mystery because empirically trying to understand them may alter our ability to let them emerge through tacit knowledge found in the unconscious mind (Polanyi 1974).

The medical model of mental health therapy puts great effort into finding symptoms for any given disorder. As mental health therapists, sometimes we need to clear our minds of analytical thinking, and simply listen to the flow of life energy between client and therapist. Believers in mindfulness have already figured this out. Phenomenologists many years ago figured this out the hard way before the advent of neuroscience. They originally entered the world of the empirically minded mental health therapists and found themselves labeled as not scientifically sound. Ironically, only recently have empirical-minded therapists found "nonthinking" a legitimate part of the therapy process. In the case study, the meaningful moments were not based on cognitive analysis but through intuition and insight. They emerged in the moment by the connections made by Peter in a visceral manner with Paul. Out of respect for those more empirical-minded readers, it was Peter's mirror neurons in his prefrontal lobe that reflected Paul's meaningful emotions and set off the intuitive responses to Paul's statements (Ladd 2018). Or, in more layperson language, it was the practice of empathy that encouraged Paul to feel comfortable in therapy and allowed him to reveal meaningful parts of his experiences. Empathy opens the door for nuances to exist, and nuances open the door for meaningful experiences to be shared. These are phenomena used by experiential therapists to work through client experiences, rather than recognizing a cluster of symptoms that justifies a disorder given by an expert.

Another example of medical model thinking is symptoms connected to verbal and nonverbal communication and behavior in a medical model. The empirical therapist takes verbal and nonverbal communication and behavior at face value. These communications or behaviors reflect empirically created symptoms that hold importance when diagnosing a patient, and these clusters of symptoms identify disorders established in a therapeutic treatment plan. In total, they add up to an empirical diagnosis that follows the patient through the process of therapy.

Experiential nuances are quite different than medical model symptoms. First in therapy, the therapist does not take these communications or behaviors at face value. They are considered gestures that fine-tune the meaning in a dialogue between therapist and client to a deeper level of meaning. The symptom of suicide ideation for chronic depression may find a different meaning according to the nuance shared by the client. The nuance of giving the therapist a "cold, hard stare" when discussing suicide ideation may intuitively stand for a client who has pre-meditatively made up his or her mind to commit suicide. If the therapist recognizes the meaning behind this nuance, it may take the dialogue between therapist and client in a different direction, possibly a discussion on "what was meaningful when you made up your mind?" As compared to a client discussing suicide ideation where the therapist has insight into frantic glances of someone who sees no way out but to commit suicide. The therapist might ask, "How can I help you look at other possibilities."

The meaning between the two may be in the first example, premeditation while in the second a frantic call for help. It may be the nuances in both of these examples have a different purpose and meaning for continuing the dialogue between both parties. Neither example is taken at face value or considered a symptom of depression. The nuances in the examples reflect the intentionality behind the client's future experiences. Such examples are difficult to understand through an empirical mind, and most likely these examples may be described as guesses or assumptions. In an experiential mind, these nuances can be intuitive, not calculated guesses or assumptions. They emerge through the meaning-making taking place in the dialogue between therapist and client. Their identity is not only an observed gesture or behavior. They are meaningful clues to possible experiences in a client's future. They are based on the skill of empathy and are revealed through the basic trust in the therapy process.

If one is looking for empirical proof of the efficacy of nuances, look no further. They are a part of each client's unique experiences, and not the empirical exactness of symptomatic behavior. Yet, regarding effectiveness, they are found in creating deep meaning in any work of art, and in any musical masterpiece, and in any therapy session where a nuance signals an "aha moment" of insight, if the therapist is skilled enough to notice them.

Over the years as a mental health therapist, the battle rages on between my empirical mind and my curious mind. Within my empirical mind, nuances do not explain anything in therapy in great detail. They seem interesting, but in the world of medical model therapy, they seem fairly insignificant phenomena. They certainly will not get client insurance reimbursement money or replace the glutinous desire for psychotropic drugs. In my curious mind that stays open to the experiences of clients, nuances will pop out unexpectedly revealing a fine-tuned meaningful experience, sometimes joyful, sometimes tragic, but nevertheless filled with wisdom and meaning. In those moments, I try not to analyze the process, instead I try to trust it. Not because I can prove it but because it works.

NOTES

1. The mature person becomes able to differentiate feelings into as many nuances, strong and passionate experiences, or delicate and sensitive ones, as in the different passages of music in a symphony. Unfortunately, many of us have feelings limited like notes in a bugle call. Rollo May, "Eleventh Annual Goodreads Choice Awards (1987)." The medical model dismisses many of the nuances that are a part of a mental health disorder—that eliminates the client going through a disorder with personal nuances that uniquely guide human suffering. Without understanding the client's nuances, suffering can be perceived as indistinguishable from one client to another.

2. "The idea comes to me from outside of me—and is like a gift. I then take the idea and make it my own—that is where the skill lies," classical composer, Johannes Brahms. https://www.goodreads.com/author/quotes/72792. Whether an actor, musician, or an artist, it is the nuances that separate these professionals from good to greatness in their unique fields. I believe, this is also the case with mental health experiential therapists. I have had the privilege of seeing Carl Rogers in action during therapy. What appeared as normal behavior to the untrained eye was filled with nuances with those who had practiced looking for them. The ability to look past the drama and observe the nuances of trauma is a skill worth practicing. Rogers's week-long visit to St. Lawrence University (Fall): 1984.

Chapter 9

Ownership versus Renter-Ship

It is important when talking about client problems that the agreed-upon solutions are owned by the client not the therapist. A medical model presents different solutions to patients. One possibility being some form of therapy technique. If the client has not taken ownership, and has not found personal meaning in the technique, the end result may be practicing it during therapy and then shortly thereafter forgetting to use it. Without personally incorporating the therapy technique into a meaningful experience, it can be overrun by previous experiences such as negative emotional patterns and bad habits especially when experiencing large traumas or ongoing chronic disorders (Richardson and Peter 2015).

Therapy techniques can be a major focus in mental health, but at what level of learning are they being presented to clients, and do different levels of learning determine their usefulness? In order to better describe, at what level clients learn therapy techniques, let us turn to Bloom's Taxonomy for clarification. The above taxonomy is well-known to professional educators, but in the field of mental health an explanation seems appropriate. I am taking the liberty of presenting an educational model of learning and using it to describe how therapists learn and apply therapy techniques in the field of mental health. Bloom's Taxonomy is a model designed to evaluate different levels of learning in any number of situations (de Beer 2017).[1]

For the sake of discussion, I will be talking about what takes place when learning a therapy technique. In figure 9.1 the learning levels of memory and comprehension show at the lower end of the taxonomy, the least-involved learning practices. When someone asks you to memorize anything, you may not even comprehend it, but if you have a good memory and you can recite it back, then you have learned it at a basic level of learning. One level up on the figure 9.1 diagram according to Bloom are those people that not only

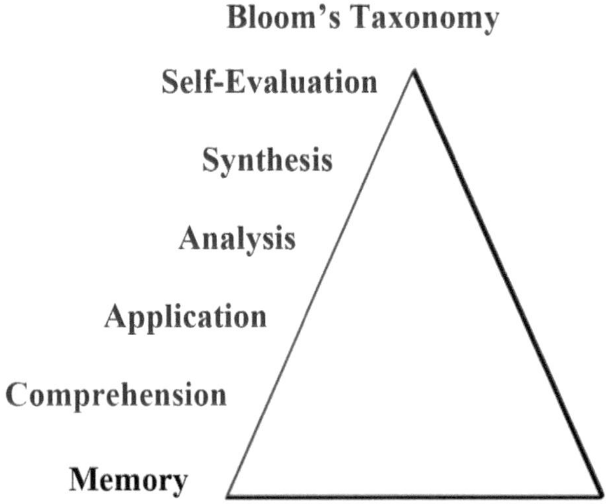

Figure 9.1 Bloom's Taxonomy.

remember what was taught but also comprehend what it means. I call this type of learning, passive learning, because it is built on passively acquiring information with little need for action or commitment. Regarding therapy techniques, at the level of memory and comprehension a patient is not required to do much, especially if they have a good memory and an adequate brain. They may sit in the therapist's office while she or he describes therapy techniques, and the clients may ask questions and try to comprehend what the therapist described to them. They may be learning something that will eventually be used as a technique in future therapy sessions. In the next visit, the therapist might ask whether they remember what they learned about the technique. Or, some curious patients may take advantage of memory and comprehension and learn through "Googling" discussed information, and then making assumptions about therapy techniques, and how to use them.

Once you ascend to the level of learning through application, on Bloom (figure 9.1), especially medical model-oriented therapists may do their best in helping patients apply therapy techniques as interventions to reduce patient suffering. At this point in my experience, patients do not have to emotionally embrace these remedies but learn to physically apply them with the hope of making therapeutic interventions that lower their symptoms. This happens not only with therapy techniques but also with psychotropic drugs. Patients do not embrace or claim ownership when taking a drug. They take them to reduce symptoms. Practicing psychological techniques or taking psychotropic drugs demonstrate success for many patients in mental health. At the application level of learning, an expert-oriented medical model therapist can help patients practice such technique as CBT, homework assignments, exposure therapy, and so on. It is a comfortable level of learning for medical model-oriented thinkers, who can control the process by clients practicing the techniques, and therapists remaining in the role of expert in the learning process.

When using medical model therapy techniques, the primary goal is whether patients comprehend how the techniques work and to successfully apply them as an intervention. Yet, I have watched medical model therapists help their patients understand and successfully apply these techniques, only when leaving therapy have them drift away in a matter of months. Sometimes patients return to previously learned, dysfunctional patterns of behavior, or they simply forget to use their newfound techniques, when they could be beneficial in any number of circumstances. In these cases, I like to use the metaphor where patients act as though they "rented" these techniques but do not "own" them. Obviously, this is not the case in many learned therapy techniques practiced in a medical model, yet in my experience, it is common enough that I must at least mention it in this chapter.

There is a different perspective when using an experiential model with therapy techniques. Experiential therapy becomes a collaborative effort where applying techniques happen at a point in the dialogue between client and therapist where a technique is added, not as an intervention but to reinforce intentionality found in the personal accomplishments by the client. For example, in trauma-informed care, a client learns the technique of EMDR after exploring and accepting the many traumas in life that led to his or her compulsive behavior. By going to higher levels of learning on Bloom's Taxonomy called analysis and synthesis, the traumas are analyzed and synthesized into different possibilities to overcome the damage caused by these traumas. Now these techniques have become a more personal phenomena. At this point, any number of therapy techniques may be learned that specifically aid the client in finding personal meaning in their traumatic experiences. Some of these learned techniques may lead to the emergence of more traumatic experiences, and more possibilities for using therapy techniques. In an experiential form of therapy, clients can take ownership of these new possibilities, and the techniques that helped them get there.

Through the meaningful and collaborative dialogue taking place in therapy, clients can reach higher levels of learning indicated on Bloom's Taxonomy (figure 9.1). Through analysis by having worked and talked through an experience, and through synthesis by making the worked through and talked through experience a personal choice toward recovery. Therapy techniques become a valuable addition to both of these endeavors. In this way, clients grow into a more closely connected relationship to these techniques. In other words, when practicing at these higher levels of learning by analyzing and synthesizing their experiences, clients can make therapy techniques their own, and not necessarily practiced as an intervention by the therapist. *When dialogue and discovery direct clients to practice a therapy technique, the intention is not formulated around an intervention to reduce symptoms but an intentional act to reinforce clients' beliefs regarding their experiences.* These techniques may become a part of client identity at these levels of learning.

Even though phenomenology (study of experience) seems less scientific and more driven by individual client intentionality, it still works at a higher level of learning when including therapy techniques than using medical model technique interventions. In therapy when client and therapist through dialogue, begin finding meaning as to why a certain therapy technique is important, a higher level of learning emerges (Kelly 2018). It is where techniques are filled with meaning-making, and not only a medical model procedure for reducing symptoms (Lacey 2006). When a client learns at the level of analysis and synthesis, on Bloom, the meaning behind any discussed experience becomes more durable and permanent.

When you practice dialogue through analysis and synthesis of personal experiences, you may also learn something about yourself. A client must become more emotionally involved with higher levels of learning, because of the personal nature when talking about these experiences (Fink 2000). Such phenomena as resilience, courage, and doubt come into play. When clients take ownership of their therapy experiences, they tend to protect them as a part of their identity. When clients "rent" techniques in therapy to reduce their symptoms, at some point in the future, they run the risk of them drifting away, with little connection to the meaningful experiences taking place in their lives.

At the top of Bloom's Taxonomy is self-evaluation, the highest level of learning. Ultimately, this is one of the aspirations embraced by experiential therapists. Empowering clients to self-evaluate and self-regulate their experiences help integrate a client into a whole person with new values and skills (Siegel 2016). When counseling techniques meet high levels of self-evaluation and self-regulation, they become a part of the meaningful experiences that create positive growth and change. For example, at some point a client who is seeking a sense a peace in his or her life may evaluate mindfulness training as an important addition to other positive experiences surrounding their sense of sought-after peace, as compared to, for example, mindfulness used as an intervention to reduce a client's anxiety without exploring the meaningful importance of how it could be connected to a client's sense of peace. The clients may reduce their anxiety through mindfulness and still not find peace.

Sometimes only reducing symptoms is one part of the experiences a client goes through in therapy. It satisfies what is learned through symptoms reduction but may fall short of satisfying the meaning-making that is learned while forming a client's beliefs and identity. In phenomenology, the power of personal choice liberates clients to accept or reject learning a therapy technique. When people choose to learn a technique in an experiential model, it is grounded in the intentionality of the client—they want to not because they need to (Ladd and Churchill 2012). Therefore, the choice goes beyond learning a counseling technique. It is a commitment to one's self that learning the technique has become a part of the experiences that define the client as a human being. It becomes a part of how one lives, and not what one needs to practice.

In a medical model, therapy techniques are used as part of a diagnosis and treatment plan. They are chosen by experts who make a judgment, a calculation that a patient will benefit from these techniques. Patients practicing techniques deemed important by the therapist may not emotionally and psychologically hold the same importance for themselves. Even when patients have made the determination that techniques will be practiced as a part of their daily experiences. Awareness of the technique and having practiced the technique is not necessarily something patients have personally embraced—unless the therapist can go to higher levels of learning where the question of "why" to use it finds meaning in the patient's everyday experiences.

It is important to remind mental health therapists that a patient's everyday experiences are filled with countless other patterns and rituals collected over the years such as trauma is always in the back of my mind, I am competent but don't feel competent, people seem to love me so why do I hate myself?, and so on. Without some form of ownership based on personal meaning, highly effective therapy techniques can be what patients want to do, but they have not reached the level of "what they think they need to do." I have discussed this phenomenon with numerous clients who place a therapy technique as their number one priority, and by the end of the month the technique has dramatically dropped in priority, or does not show up on the daily radar at all.

Experiential therapists are not immune from client enthusiasm evaporating after learning therapy techniques that have been occasionally practiced over time. Techniques may find a way down the priority list of client's everyday experiences. Furthermore, having clients practice techniques during therapy is a different phenomenon than when practicing them, for example, two months later. Experiences may have changed, and what was of high priority in therapy is bumped to a lower priority, without any conscious decision on the part of the former client. This may be why therapy techniques for the experiential therapist are usually not considered useful before establishing a therapeutic alliance. The therapy that follows a therapeutic alliance is based on collaborative dialogue where a therapy technique can become attached to meaningful changes in a client's life.

A client with overwhelming anxiety does not want her children to see her cry because she believes it will upset them. After establishing a therapeutic alliance, the dialogue has revealed how meaningful this experience holds in the client's everyday life. This experience is not only attached to relieving anxiety but also affects her relationship with her children. Now, for example, the technique of *slow shallow breathing* has meaning more than simply a skill to deal with her symptoms of anxiety. It becomes something she attaches to meaningful encounters with her children. It now shifts into a more purposeful experience by taking ownership of the technique by attaching it to the strong, meaningful connection she has with her children. In this manner, the therapy technique becomes a part of her life story with her children, and not only a reduction in symptoms.

When people sign up for mental health workshops, seminars, and online courses they already have an intention to learn some form of psychological information, including therapy techniques. Again, according the intentionality behind learning this information will determine whether the learner takes ownership of this information or is he or she just renting it for the sake of awareness. A point to consider in mental health therapy depends on the level of learning one wants to pursue. At lower levels of learning, I believe that therapy techniques run the risk of remaining only information.

I also believe that most educational opportunities in mental health stay at the level of comprehension. Others offer learning at the application level through role plays and other activities. It becomes an occasional occurrence when educational information outside of actual mental health therapy begins working at the level of analysis, synthesis, and self-evaluation. Learning at these levels requires a personal risk of one's self. It may require a vulnerability to learn meaningful experiences that may have been concealed for years. At these levels of learning, therapy techniques almost need to be attached to some meaningful experience in one's personal life. The therapy technique then ceases to be the focus of attention, but a method to fortify through learning a skill that strengthens the intentionality of the client (Ladd 2018).

CASE STUDY

The university was noted for having a strong graduate mental health counseling program that spanned two years. During the second year, each graduate student was required to fulfill an internship in a mental health clinic, hospital, or a university counseling center. At a neighboring university, their counseling center agreed to take one of the better graduate students from the program. Janis agreed to use the neighboring counseling center as her internship requirement. Up till this point, she had a highly productive experience, and showed a great deal of compassion and empathy in her style of counseling.

In the beginning days of her internship at the counseling center, she was told that one of the requirements was that she use CBT as her method for treating her clients. At first, she showed no resistance to this, because it was one of the techniques that she was most familiar, and she had extensive practice in performing the technique. About a month into her internship at a staff meeting, she was criticized for not using the technique with all her clients. She was informed that her treatment plans were falling behind, and she needed to show proof that her clients were receiving the proper care. The rationale behind using CBT was that it had been proven effective more than most other therapy techniques, and it had the research to back up its effectiveness. She agreed to use it even though, she believed, some of the experiences of her clients were not exactly fitting for the technique.

The fortunate part, at least she thought, was her clients put up little resistance to learning and using the technique. However, she slowly believed that the technique was taking up most of her time with clients without getting to know their underlying experiences in any great detail. This was troubling, for her compassion and empathy seemed to be pushed to the side, and she felt it in the relationship with her clients. Even though they showed a level of compliance in learning the technique, she worried about the lack of forming a therapeutic alliance between them. When this was brought up at a staff meeting the group emphasized that they were a CBT-oriented counseling center, and she needed to improve her willingness to practice at the high standards set out by the staff.

After much thought and some highly felt discussions with other internship students, she approached her supervisor with a problem. She told Yasmeen, her supervisor, that it was important to follow the guidelines of the counseling center, but she found herself slowly becoming distant from her clients, and increasingly becoming a problem with other staff members. She also described the emotional upheaval in herself, as tears ran down her face during the description she shared with Yasmeen. This was quite a shock for Yasmeen who believed she was one of the finer students in the program and that it was important to immediately discuss this situation with the counseling center's chief supervisor.

The meeting between Yasmeen and the internship's chief supervisor can only be described as unpleasant. The supervisor wanted to know at what level of training was the graduate school sending out students who did not seem to comply with the guidelines explained to them in the internship's beginning orientation. Janis was couched as a highly noncompliant student who questioned the procedures at the counseling center and seemed to resist the research on CBT. Yasmeen, in attempting to be fair, commented that Janis would like more time to establish a therapeutic alliance with her clients, and that not all of them fit within the boundaries where one would use CBT.

The counseling center's supervisor took great offense to this statement and wondered whether Janis was the right fit for what was happening with the rest of the staff. Yasmeen made a quick intuitive decision that Janis was not going to get a fair supervised experience, and told the supervisor, "I agree. I do not believe she is a good fit at your counseling center and I will be making a change in her assignment. Thank you for your time." The supervisor was again offended and showed Yasmeen to the door. As she was driving back to the graduate school, she made a note to not use that counseling center again. She concluded that the problem had very little to do with the effectiveness of CBT but more of a problem with the staff's inflexible attitude for recognizing the many other facets involved in human experience.

When Yasmeen talked to Janis, she was relieved but obviously had her confidence shaken, and the placement Yasmeen was considering did not make her confidence grow any stronger. Yasmeen wanted to place her in a nearby psychiatric hospital that had a program for sexual offenders. Janis thought, "If I cannot make it with college students, how will I ever make it with this group?" Yasmeen asked Janis to trust her, even though she had strong reservations about the placement. However, what Janis found was the freedom to meet these patients at their level of disfunction, where she had the opportunity to build an alliance with them, and eventually use the most noted compassion and empathy where she stood out in her graduate education. The irony in all of this was that with certain patients she eventually used CBT.

DISCUSSION

The case study reinstates the old argument between efficacy and effectiveness. In a medical model of mental health therapy there is great value placed on the efficacy of a therapy technique (Daniels and Larsen 2001). Yet, the term efficacy signifies studies under more controlled conditions where experts test for positive changes in patient behavior, and these changes are backed by high levels of accurate statistical probability. Effectiveness refers to more pragmatic, real-life conditions where an efficacious therapy technique either works or it does not work based on the experiences taking place in real-life settings (Chorpita, Becker and Daleiden 2007). In evaluating mental health-oriented therapy techniques, efficacy refers more to the techniques themselves, while effectiveness references to the real-life experiences that clients go through.

In medical model mental health therapy much of what is valued pertains to, for example, the efficacy of the diagnosis, the efficacy of the cluster of designated symptoms backing the diagnosis, and in this case, the efficacy of techniques used in mental health therapy. The emphasis on the techniques used coincides with a model that begins with a hypotheses (diagnosis), based on a cluster of symptoms, and ends with a treatment plan to reduce these symptoms (Beidas and Kendall 2010). Therapy techniques under these assumptions are given the highest priority, and the plethora of techniques available speaks to the importance given to them. In the case study, the counseling program at the university where Janis was an intern was acutely focused on the therapy technique of CBT. Their understanding was established on the efficacy of a technique that had proven itself to reduce client symptoms.

Their counseling center's dogmatic belief in techniques is not unfamiliar to experiential therapists. In order to be an expert, one needs expert-level techniques even though techniques are responsible for very low efficacy in making changes during mental health therapy (Hansen 2018). What has been proven efficacious is the establishment of a therapeutic alliance between client and therapist (Hansen 2018). Establishing a therapeutic alliance is not one of the immediate directions taken with an expert-oriented mental health therapist. In my opinion, very few experts practicing classic medical model mental health therapy focus on their humanity when connecting with clients. They tend to focus on their expertise. They may be the more experiential therapists who encourage collaborative, intimate, and real-life dialogue during the therapy experience. Certain conditions to capture one's humanity come to mind. Conditions as described by icons such as Carl Rogers and Viktor Frankl emphasize humanity as a fundamental concept when doing mental health therapy. Rogers reiterated the practice of positive regard, empathy, and genuineness, and with Frankl, selfless acts, an appreciation for meaning, and a commitment to loving others became an emphasis in the therapy process (Rogers 1980; Frankl 2014). These are not necessarily defined as techniques, but expressions of one's humanity, and are at the heart of establishing a therapeutic alliance in therapy. Such humanistic themes can be considered efficacious but are better described as effective within the experience between client and therapist. Experiential therapists, within their search for avenues of possibilities for their clients, rely more on human values, and not necessarily therapy techniques to achieve client growth and change.

In the case study, Janis did not work from a technique-oriented expertise. She saw clients through the eyes of human beings that wanted a connection with her. She had no problem believing in the technique of CBT. Her problem at the expert-oriented counseling center was her greater belief in the human connection she valued between herself and her clients. When she was placed in a different setting, and one could argue a more difficult setting and with more egregious clients, she made those connections. After establishing a therapeutic alliance, she and one client agreed to try CBT as a technique that may help bolster client confidence in the client's journey toward growth and change. In this case, she was not working from a model that promoted efficacious techniques. She chose a model that allowed her to be creative in the dialogue she was having with not just this specific client but all of her clients.

The term "phenomenology" depicts the study of experience. Experiential therapists do not see themselves as experts but as collaborators who are willing to travel along with clients on their journey to explore effective possibilities for their lives. In this regard, it is not about the technique, or the diagnosis, or the symptoms. It is about the experience. Simply put, how can I as an experiential therapist help the client work through negative experiences and guide them into a position where they can make positive changes to their lives? How do I make the experience the problem, and not the client? How do I accept labels, diagnoses, efficacious therapy techniques for the *business* of mental health, while focusing in therapy on the client's experiences? These are the questions surrounding the experiential therapist.

The issues of ownership versus renter-ship of therapy techniques are one of the many issues that define the philosophical stance taken in experiential mental health therapy. In a client's experience, to learn a technique for the purpose of reducing symptoms may never find the powerful meaning connected to personal experiences. What is put into perspective for the experiential therapist is the connection between therapy techniques and the meaningful experiences of the clients. The focus now is not on the technique but on whether the technique will be effective in helping the client make changes to his or her life experiences.

Can the client claim ownership of the technique as a part of a personal life story, or is the technique only a rental that is practiced in good faith until the life story overwhelms the client with old dysfunctional patterns of behavior? From an experiential perspective, either the technique becomes a part of a client's life story or it does not. Meaning-making is about each person's unique experiences through life, where some hold more weight than others. Practicing techniques for mental health experts may hold less weight than practicing them for one's self.

To understand the value of techniques in therapy, it must be traced back to what was learned while practicing a therapy technique. Was that technique learned, according to Bloom, at the levels of comprehension and application where the client understood and practiced to the satisfaction of an expert, or was it learned at levels of analysis, synthesis, and self-evaluation, where it was integrated into client experiences at a level of importance, not by an expert but by the client. Sometimes in experientially oriented therapy, it becomes important to trust the client's ability to learn whether a technique is valuable or not. Without forming a therapeutic alliance this becomes a difficult phenomenon to accomplish.

As someone who has taught techniques of counseling for many years, I do not take these words lightly. Realization of different counseling techniques and their importance have not escaped my perspective. Yet, I also realize the importance of forming a therapeutic alliance with clients, not as an expert but as a collaborator. A therapist who is willing to hear the client's story and accepts the value of their experiences becomes more closely united as a human being beyond the client/therapist relationship. We have survived on this planet for thousands of years, not on using the most efficacious technique for survival but on talking to each other, and coming to some form of agreement as to what techniques, strategies, and plans of action will most effectively address the experiences before us. We are indeed individuals, but we are also components within larger social systems that take on identities of their own (Wooley 2015). The connection between therapist and client is one of those socially connected identities. In my opinion, phenomenological intentionality is the connection between client and therapist, and will yield more effective results than the intentions held only by an efficaciously oriented expert. This belief requires mental health therapy to also acknowledge the client and his or her experiences as the *unrecognized experts* in this process (Ladd and Churchill 2012).

It is only clients who can own counseling techniques instead of renting them, not the therapist. No harm is done at lower levels of learning as demonstrated in Bloom's Taxonomy regarding comprehension and application, when thinking about therapy techniques. Medical model therapists work at this level of teaching techniques to clients most of the time. This also stands for workshops, online, and in-house therapy technique courses, and other activities that surround comprehension and application methods of learning. When therapy techniques reach the level of analysis, synthesis, and self-evaluation on Bloom, the learning becomes highly personal and emotionally significant to the client. We are now asking clients how they analyze these techniques for themselves, and how do they want to synthesize them into their life experiences, and do they want them to be a part of how they evaluate themselves.

I have a friend who practices techniques of mindfulness every day not based on how it relieves negative symptoms of stress but how it helps reinforces his belief in living a life that minimizes stress. He finds meaning in living a meaningful life, not on techniques that reduce stress. In a medical model with an exceptionally talented therapist, therapy techniques can be raised to higher levels of learning, and some of my colleagues are examples of this achievement. So, the emphasis is not directed to the abilities of mental health therapists. It is more directed to the procedures found when practicing in a system, as in the traditional medical model, where comprehension and application of therapy techniques seem enough in reducing patient symptoms.

In contemporary mental health culture, the experiential therapist is faced with numerous challenges. Shall they approach therapy as an expert or as a collaborator? What is important during therapy, knowledge or wisdom? Should they use neuroscience to comprehend human experience, or is it strictly knowledge that helps understand connections between the brain and the mind? Is there a difference between dialogue and discussion, and how to recognize the difference? Do we need to focus on experiential patterns, or are psychological labels enough as an indicator of effective diagnosis? Should we be more concerned with the momentum demonstrated in the therapy process, or should we rely on standardized procedures for the best possible results? Finally, should we rent out therapy techniques, or should we make sure that clients decide to own them before practicing techniques during therapy? There are no right or wrong answers to these questions, only a choice of perspective. Any legitimate profession needs alternatives to choose from. One choice is the medical model form of mental health therapy. The other alternative is an experiential model. One model comes into play when deciding on a technique controlled by efficacious data, and the other is putting trust in a technique that adds clarity and commitment to human experience.

NOTE

1. I have found that there is a close correlation between Bloom's Taxonomy and Maslow's Hierarchy of Needs when engaging in talk therapy. (Maslow came up with a hierarchy of what we need as human beings. At lower levels are physical and safety needs. Beyond these we need a sense of belonging and self-esteem. At the highest level is self-actualization.) It may be important to gain traction on Maslow's Hierarchy of Needs at least at the "Belonging Level" on Maslow before attempting to go to higher levels of analysis and synthesis on Bloom's Taxonomy in mental health therapy. "I don't care how much you know, until I know how much you care" (Ladd 2019) applies to mental health therapy. In experiential therapy, the therapeutic alliance assures that client learning fulfills the needs found on Maslow, before entering the arena of knowledge found on Bloom. Peter Ladd. 2019. "PowerPoint Presentation on Phenomenology," *YouTube Presentation*, St. Lawrence University, November 30, 2018.

Chapter 10

Flexibility versus Order

Medical model therapists work within a system that is based on order and procedures. There is a standardized set of rules that pertains to all patients seeking their help: intake, diagnosis, treatment planning, and technique administration. The experiential therapist may struggle under such order. Each client's experiences are different, so the approach taken must have flexibility to be effective. The experiential therapist believes that flexibility inspires hope. Order looks for reliability and validity. Flexibility means staying in the present moment when having a dialogue with clients. It requires being conscious of what the situation is calling for, sometimes it is helping to change client behavior, or possibly helping a client understand his or her belief system. This means being more flexible in whatever way the therapy session is going and for many clients is viewed as more valuable regarding human experience. A session could start out focusing on a client's anxiety, and end with a change in focus, possibly with a client's sense of loss. This is not the direction taken in a medical model form of mental health therapy. One way to describe it in therapy is order is win/lose, either you are right about the diagnosis or you are not. Flexibility is win/win or until you win. If the dialogue does not uncover the meaning behind the actual experience you change focus until it does.

The medical model with its formats, procedures, and standardized set of diagnoses places therapy in the position of being correct about a diagnosis, or not being correct. If not correct, the "domino effect" may happen where one decision ripples its influences on treatment plans, therapy techniques, and insurance required labels. There may be a tendency to stay with an original diagnosis rather than start over again. What also can happen is another diagnosis is added to cover up what was missing in the original diagnosis (Cherry 2019). If the original diagnosis is far off track, a patient could end up with four or five different diagnoses. I know of an Iraqi veteran who was emotionally paralyzed with PTSD but refused to quit his job in support of his family. His medical model psychiatrist instead of commending him for his resilience gave him another label of obsessive-compulsive disorder based on the psychiatrist's belief that working would increase pressure and anxiety on his symptoms of PTSD, and his refusal to stop working demonstrated his obsessive-compulsive tendencies. Later, when working with an experientially oriented therapist, he declared that working to support his family was the main reason that he survived, regarding thoughts of suicide. This example may not stand for common procedures based on keeping order in a medical model form of mental health therapy, but it makes the point that flexibility may be called for when listening to the thoughts, feelings, and behaviors of clients.

From an experiential perspective, flexibility can become vitally important in therapy during the interactions between client and therapist. The more the therapist is flexible with changes in the direction of therapy, the more a client can make the decision to change (Ladd 2018). In my experience, changing the diagnosis, treatment plan, and therapy techniques can become a major ordeal for the medical model mental health therapist, even though the patient may greatly benefit from a change in direction. This may be one reason that experiential therapists see themselves as collaborators rather than experts. Collaborators in experiential therapy are more open to change than experts, though sometimes criticized for not having a therapy plan in the beginning of therapy that emanates from their expertise. Try responding to an insurance company that is considering reimbursement for a mental health diagnosis with "I don't know yet." This may give you an idea of the unethical temptation for submitting a false narrative, or a diagnosis that smacks of vagary that could stand for just about anything.

In my opinion, unfortunately experientially oriented therapists are not rewarded for their wisdom but for their knowledge. Wisdom in mental health therapy becomes a more complicated phenomenon to understand. It is not solely based on one's training, memory, comprehension, and adherence to the norms and guidelines of the APA, though these issues are important—and it is not necessarily what clients are looking for during therapy. It is obtained through experience, education, and practice that one uses in the world, and because of this, wisdom is more about the discretion and flexibility for change when it is needed in real-life experiences (Tiberious 2008). This could not be more important than the flexibility needed when clients make crucial changes in the direction taken during therapy. From experiential thinking, it becomes more important that clients and therapists have the flexibility to change course in therapy, than whether a diagnosis is followed in an orderly fashion throughout the therapy process. Without a balance between flexibility and order, in therapy, very little wisdom seems possible.

Flexibility in therapy is also supported neurologically. One of the most focused on elements of mental health disorders for patients is the decision made by experts to take psychotropic drugs. Even more inflexible phenomena as schizophrenia or bipolar disorders through psychotropic drugs and mental health therapy mitigate some neuropathway function, though not all of them (Brown 2012). For more common mental disorders such as anxiety and depression, one of the goals is to alter habitual neuropathways in the brain such as anxiety and depression, so that feeling anxious or depressed can have meaning and purpose. Ironically, medical model mental health is more flexible in changing ineffective psychotropic drugs to fit the patient's diagnosis, than changing the diagnosis to fit the patient's experience. At least, that is my opinion.

As stated in chapter 6, "Patterns versus Labels," therapists have more flexibility in helping to change experiential patterns regarding a client's negative experiences than changing diagnostic labels reflecting a client's psychological symptoms. Sometimes mental health therapy can be a sloppy endeavor from an experiential viewpoint. The calculations provided by the medical model mental health therapist do not reflect standard operating procedures as found in medical model *physical medicine*. In physical medicine, it is much easier to standardize treatment into orderly procedures, whether it is treatment for a broken leg or treatment for heart failure.

In reality, many of the procedures in physical medicine need to be standardized and orderly or establishing an expertise in these fields can be questionable. In mental health therapy, in order to establish an expertise, sometimes client experiences have to be standardized such as found in the DSM. The attempt to standardize human experience may be the very reasons that experiential patterns make more sense than statistically driven labels. If the experience begins to change in therapy, so do attempts to describe the experiential patterns begin to change. In medical model mental health therapy, order wins the day over flexibility, even though common sense and experienced therapists would remind us that when doing therapy with clients, being flexible is a major concern, especially when orderly procedures are not in synch with human experience.

In experiential therapy, client and therapist use dialogue to freely express their ideas about a particular topic. This can be considered as a positive way of obtaining new knowledge, and also learning to accept each other's flexible points of view. Without a certain amount of flexibility in the dialogue, freedom of expression is gone. Introducing more order may turn therapy into a discussion about how to solve mental health problems where the therapist is designated the "fixer" of these problems. In my experience, medical model therapists are open to discussion rather than dialogue. In a discussion, arriving at a decision is a key component which fits more readily with a therapy process based on making judgments on a proper diagnosis, treatment planning, psychotropic drug prescriptions, and techniques for one's treatment plans. This sequence of events helps to maintain order during the medical model therapy process, but I believe this lacks the flexibility needed in dialogue where most of the moments where clients begin to make positive change materialize out of a free-flowing exchange of ideas.

Free-flowing dialogue also creates the type of flexibility therapists need in noticing subtle nuances connected to each dialogue in therapy. In a manner of speaking, nuances are not usually revealed when focusing on fulfilling a treatment plan, or when practicing a therapy technique. Nuances may need the flexibility practiced in unencumbered intuitive thinking to reveal themselves. In free-flowing dialogue, one gesture or one change in the tone of voice may trigger a shift in meaning for the client or the therapist. Without the ability to stay focused on the "real-time" dialogue taking place, such meaningful moments can be missed. For the medical model mental health therapist, moment-to-moment nuances may seem far too mystical a phenomenon than looking for symptoms that help to prove a diagnosis or give direction to a therapy session. For example, the symptom of over-expressive language by the client may signal to the therapist that the client is catastrophizing, and recommends the therapy technique of CBT, while not realizing such expressive language is a nuanced expression of the client's culture. In this example, symptoms win out over nuances. Without finding flexibility and meaning in the dialogue between client and therapist these types of nuances are unfortunately missed. I have had the privilege of working on a Native American Reservation for many years, and the number of nuances missed by beginning therapists is worth noting. In my experience, sometimes nuances are confused with symptoms unless there is flexibility in the dialogue between both parties in mental health therapy. This is especially true with cultural nuances, for example, not giving eye contact by a client may be a nuance of showing respect, instead a symptom described as loss of pleasure, connected to chronic depression. This leads to my strong belief that a client's specific culture creates meaningful nuances that remain more accurate than a cluster of medical model symptoms.

Hope is about the future having an impact on the present, while considering what has happened in the past. Hope connects the past, present, and future in a new creative way. In this regard, I believe that hope is highly transformative, possibly life-changing. Such moments in therapy are impossible to empirically measure without the flexibility to change directions when a client's life experiences find new energy and new direction—a direction with purpose and meaning. Subsequently in mental health therapy, old-mold, orderly procedures may not be considered the flexible starting point for client to capture subtle moments of hope.

Without flexibility it is hard to visualize the hope that some successful clients experience when suddenly the direction of therapy changes and new hope for the future becomes overwhelmingly clear. In experiential therapy, one of the main reasons for practicing flexibility in therapy is to create a climate of hope through client empowerment. The medical model focuses on remission of symptoms, but in experiential therapy those symptoms are not ignored but put into perspective. Symptoms, disorders, and labels are viewed by a more idealistic experiential therapist as possible roadblocks to a client's future filled with hope. There are procedures in mental health therapy that reduce symptoms of disorders in an orderly fashion, but seeing a reduction of symptoms in mental health as the main issue does not include the flexibility needed in client experiences to create a sense of hope. Without hope, remission of symptoms in therapy may not have the flexibility to change the direction in a client's life. In many cases, it allows the same direction to prevail only with less pain and suffering.

CASE STUDY

Matt was diagnosed with depression ten years ago after a serious car accident where one of his friends was killed, and he was injured. It was not guilt behind the accident that seemed the cause of the depression, nor did he lose control of his feelings. It was not even depression that ultimately was responsible for his suffering. Nevertheless, he was treated for depression through psychotropic drugs and CBT, yet ten years later not much change had taken place, until one of his friends pointed out that fact to him. His friend said, "Matt you really have not changed much over the years. You talk about the accident as though it was yesterday." Hearing this from his friends, Matt decided to talk with someone, but not about his depression, but more about not letting go of stories about the accident. He met with Caroline, a mental health counselor with more humanistic tendencies. Caroline made Matt feel comfortable by listening to his story without trying to figure out what was wrong with him. Matt described his diagnosis of depression but also told of his friend's comments about how little change was taking place in his life. Caroline pointed out to Matt that he had made a change. By listening to friends, Caroline explained that he had shifted to giving another look to the experiences that he had gone through, especially focusing on the car accident. She pointed out how important it was to have friends that help out when they see something not working in one's life, and how much he must mean to them.

After this conversation with Caroline, Matt realized that he had a choice, to continue with his belief that he was chronically depressed, or to reconsider that other answers to his mood were available, if he chose to talk about them. And, he did talk about them, with Caroline being his guide through the dialogue he presented at each meeting in therapy. At one point, he seemed to believe that maybe he was not depressed but more apathetic after Caroline demonstrated that with depression one cares too much and with apathy one cares too little. From this conversation, he realized that it was not that he cared too much about the accident. It was more based on him not wanting to do anything about it yet remaining depressed or now possibly apathetic. He knew that at times he felt emotionally numb even when engaged in sexual activity. He described in therapy as living in a bubble, present but emotionally not there. Matt also described that sometimes he would run to this bubble when overwhelming stress began to kick in. Caroline commented that it seems like your bubble has a dual purpose. On the one hand, it has affected your life in such a negative way that you have been labeled with depression, but on the other hand, it is a place to retreat when life becomes too difficult to face directly. Caroline continued, "Matt on the one hand you say that caring too much is scary, and you are much more comfortable caring too little, which does not accurately fit the description of depression, but more of apathy. You admit being more distant at times than feeling only numb as a symptom of apathy. Yet, you also have said that you avoid your feelings in stressful situations such as when having sex or sharing your feelings with friends. Matt, I do not know what you really feel when coming out of that bubble, but it is something to think about."

Between the next session Matt had an epiphany as he walked his dog in a nearby field. It was even with friends and lovers he still felt detached. After sharing this with Caroline, she said, "Now that makes sense. There is a term in trauma work called dissociation, where one protects one's self by becoming numb to any similar situation to the former experience of trauma. By closing down emotionally, are you trying to live a normal life free of the vulnerability when emotionally experiencing meaningful moments in life?" Matt said, "That is absolutely what I am doing, and do you want to know the experience I am most seeking, feeling at home. I am not depressed but very homesick, if that makes any sense, even though I am with my friends and lovers constantly." Caroline replied, "Matt when you go back into that bubble of dissociation are you physically with them, but emotionally in a distant place?"

It took Matt a few weeks to think about and describe his homesickness to Caroline, but at one point he stated that he had to do something about it. Caroline softly stated, "What do you want to do?" The next week Matt came back to the therapy session looking exhausted, but lighter around his eyes and seemed to flow in a more rhythmic way. Caroline asked, "Wow! You seem different." Matt told her that after inviting his friends and lover to dinner and that after dinner was over he spontaneously broke down and cried and said that he was homesick, and he needed their help. One of his friends said, "Welcome home!" He thanked all of them for hanging in there with him over the years, and he will try to remain more emotionally human with their help. They all laughed and welcomed him back one more time.

On return to therapy with Caroline, he asked her to explain what had gone on in his therapy that brought him to this vulnerable but wonderful place in his life. She described his experience to him as though it was a story with the beginning being his diagnosis of depression to the point when friends called him out when not getting better. She further said, "We both at one point talked about maybe it was apathy because you seemed to be avoiding life, not intensely upset that life was passing you by." She said, "The story continued when our discussion turned to how you at a certain stressful point would go emotionally numb as though you were in a bubble. You were there but not emotionally there. All I did was give that type an experience a name, dissociation, though that may be the least important point in the whole experience. What was important is how you would go in and out of the bubble, but not really connecting emotionally with friends or loved ones. Eventually, I simply asked if you knew what to call the emotion that you were avoiding, and an epiphany happened when you realized it was homesickness. Finally, you decided to deal with your homelessness by telling your friends, and then it all spilled out in a fountain of tears. I tried not to tell you what to do or advise you in a direction that I thought you should go. You seemed empowered enough to figure that out on your own, and you did, and because you did, you were the person who changed the direction of your personal life, story."

Matt said to Caroline, "If I get caught again can I come back and have further conversations?" Caroline said,

> "Of course, but you are at a point where the conversations between friends and lovers seem to be the direction you are headed. The important part of the therapy was the collaboration between you and your friends, including me, and your willingness to remain flexible as your experiences unfolded. Regarding depression, I would call it dissociation but more importantly is you being able see the pattern of going in and out of your bubble, and how the bubble has protected you from the trauma, but also at the expense of being unable to have emotional feelings, or to feel at home (Buckley 1974). When you could finally come out emotionally, the bubble became less of a factor. On the other hand, if you want to go all the way back to the trauma from the accident, and how it led you to protect yourself from the emotional trauma, I am willing to also go back with

you, but that is your decision. Regardless of whether we go back or not, you have found a new avenue to travel for a more emotionally filled future."

DISCUSSION

One of the first criticisms that may come out is that Matt never went back and was debriefed from the original accident and found out how it influenced his life. From a trauma-informed care perspective, if what was meaningful to him was to go back, then some form of working through the accident would be appropriate. Matt's friends wanted their friend back home, and it was at this point that his story took on meaning. This is one of the many reasons as to why flexibility in therapy remains such an important phenomenon for the experiential therapist. The more structured therapist might through some debriefing protocol go back to the accident and try to have Matt share the experience of the original trauma. Yet the original trauma was not where Matt was at in his mind. He had resolved the impact of the car accident by developing a pattern of disassociation. Sometimes, dissociation is seen only as a mental health disorder, however, in the case of Matt it acted as a solution to Matt's inability after the accident to deal with his emotions. The problem came more from his friends than from Matt. They noticed little change even though he had gone to a therapist and received psychotropic drugs. In essence, they jarred him out of his dissociation to the point where he could feel again, along with the help of Caroline who set the stage for this to happen. Without flexibility he may have settled on depression as a state of mind that he would live with for the foreseeable future, and still suffer from homesickness.

In medical model mental health therapy, the diagnosis is reached after symptoms of a patient are established, and right before the creation a treatment plan. In an experiential model, as Carl Jung has stated, "Maybe diagnosis should come at the end of therapy not the beginning" (Jung 2003). We may have become a solution-oriented society who looks for quick, clear solutions, especially some people who enter as patients into the mental health system. Sometimes, they are given solutions when the professionals still do not know the problem. In the case of Matt this *was* the problem. When he realized how he was coping with his previous trauma by dissociating, it finally led him to his real problem of not feeling at home. He was not depressed, even though there were symptoms evident of depression. He was not apathetic, even though his emotional bubble let him act as if he cared while staying in a safe place. The vulnerability of losing anyone else through an accident or otherwise was now protected. In the end, the discovery was that he emotionally missed his friends and lovers. Through the help of Caroline setting the stage for him at each awareness and opportunity for change, Matt had the flexibility to shift gears to discover new things about himself. To work through a traumatic experience, not by the help of an expert but through the wisdom found in true dialogue that demonstrated the flexibility needed in the healing process. By allowing the nuances in the dialogue between them to show direction and to create hope, his curious mind kept seeking out an answer. The focus was on the traumatic pattern. We could call it euphemistically the "In-and-Out-of-the-Bubble Pattern": that he was using to survive his original trauma, that allowed him to emotionally close down, but at the same time, continue his life in a fairly normal existence.

In dealing with trauma, the above story is not unfamiliar to the mental health therapists who have an understanding not only of phenomenology but also of trauma-informed care, a movement that begins with experience, rather than with personal disorders. The five principles of trauma-informed care are safety, choice, collaboration, trustworthiness, and empowerment (Tello 2019). Trauma-informed care as demonstrated in the case study is at its foundation an experiential method. As seen throughout this book with other experiential methods of giving therapy to clients, trauma-informed care shifts the focus from "What's wrong with you?" to "What happened to you?" Again, we see a different approach to mental disorders by emphasizing client experiences over client disorders; trauma-informed care also recognizes that traditional service approaches can re-traumatize consumers and family members. Additionally, trauma-informed care is a person-centered response focused on improving an individual's all-around wellness, rather than simply treating symptoms of mental illness. Here are four guidelines that earmark trauma-informed care (Kezelmann and Stavropoulos 2012):

Compassion and Dependability—when we experience compassionate and dependable relationships, we reestablish trusting connections with others that foster mutual wellness.

Collaboration and Empowerment—when we are prepared for and given real opportunities to make choices for ourselves and our care, we feel empowered and can promote our own wellness.

Resilience and Recovery—when we focus on our strengths and have clear steps we can take toward wellness, we are more likely to be resilient and recover.

Safety and Security—when we can create a safe and secure environment for others, we help find meaning in one's own wellness.

Combine these guidelines and with the experiential themes found in the chapters of this book, you are on your way to understanding an experiential thinker. This is not intended to discredit the work of medical model mental health therapists but to make the mental health profession more holistic and flexible. Client/patients should be given an orientation on both medical models and experiential models and be allowed the flexibility to choose the direction they would like to take in therapy—either reduce symptoms or help become a more fully functioning human being. Up until a number of years ago there was little choice. If you were suffering from a mental disorder, then it had to be treated and fixed much as in the procedures used in physical medicine. If a choice is not what you should be giving client/patients then at least offer all models that can be sequentially used, beginning with a reduction in symptoms followed by the development of resilience and hope. Yet, without a certain flexibility of choice, the institutions found in mental health will make that choice for you.[1]

I have pointed out the trauma-informed care model as having made the choice to be more experiential and recovery-oriented than symptoms-reduction, symptoms maintenance-oriented therapy: focusing on trauma as one way that experiential thinkers can practice their beliefs and still be accepted by mainstream institutions. It may be that the time has come for a more diversified set of procedures to practice in helping people with their mental problems. Even therapy techniques may also have a choice to work in a medical model set of orderly procedures or be used during the flexibility found in dialogue where the therapy techniques support the meaning behind the dialogue. This is a more adjunct role where these techniques stop being used as interventions based not on dialogue but through guesses of probability that tend to ignore one's personal experiences.

Unfortunately, flexibility is becoming more problematic in the field of mental health. Experiential thinkers depend on the flexibility in dialogue to collaborate with clients and move in a direction wherever their personal experiences take them. However, with the constant attempt to medicalize mental health culture, experiential thinkers are being threatened emotionally and psychologically by some of the inflexible mandates handed down by the standardization found in mental health facilities and managed care programs. There is nothing wrong with finding mental health experts who will guide us. However, not at the expense of meaningful dialogue where successful outcomes depend on both client and therapist (Ladd 2018).[2] The flexibility needed to conduct a more experiential form of therapy, hopefully validates the importance of dialogue between human beings as a fundamental building block in our society, and in the field of mental health. Bonding together through flexible meaningful dialogue is a part of our social makeup and possibly our survival.

NOTES

1. "The curious paradox is that when I accept myself just as I am, then I can change." Carl Rogers and John Wood. 1974. *Client-Centered Theory*. Oxford: Brunner/Mazel.

2. The medical model therapist consumed with symptom reduction spends most of the time relieving symptoms that contain thoughts, behavior, and feelings. An experiential therapist focuses on identity, and based on finding it, making thoughts, behavior, and feelings easier to change. There is little sense in changing symptoms that cannot withstand the power of one's beliefs and identity. For me, mental health therapy is primarily about identity change.

Chapter 11

Dwelling (Attending) versus Rumination

Much of what happens during medical model therapy is to focus on a patient's pathology. Experiential therapists make no preconceived focus. During the process of creating a therapeutic alliance, and helping clients work through their experiences, the therapeutic process used is based on intentionality. It is the ability of individuals to link their inner consciousness and perceptions with their outer purposes and actions (Schmit 1994). The degree to which people accomplish this linkage is a measure of the intensity of their intentionality. Intentionality is consciousness actively reaching out toward the object in a *directed* way (Hockaday, Purkey, and Davis 2001). It provides a structure which gives experience meaning. Human capacity for intentionality has great value for therapists and their clients. By raising the internal clarity of intentionality, individuals are more likely to direct their behavior in healthy and productive ways (May 1965). For example, a client has a clear vision of how to turn around his alcoholic lifestyle and is taking steps to make the change.

In therapy, intentionality is when the client shares his or her experiences, and the therapist and client find purpose and meaning in future possibilities emerging during therapy (Ladd 2012). Intentionality is based on consciously finding meaning in life's projects (Ladd 2009). In experiential therapy, one of the purposes of intentionality is to *attend to something meaningful*. This could be a project, a person, a cause, and so on. Conversely, in a medical model, the intent is on one's pathology, which keeps the focus on the patient's disorder and mostly on the patient's past. Here is where a patient can fall into the trap of rumination of constantly analyzing experiences over and over again (Barron 2012). Rumination has a tendency to worsen the negative and, I believe, is one of the flaws associated with a pathology-focused medical model. Intentionality through attending in experiential therapy has a tendency to give meaning inside one's self and with purpose outside of one's self.

One of the practices that clients use to meet purpose and meaning in their intentionality is to use the concept of "dwelling." Dwelling is focusing on a possibility for the future but not through analysis, but through attending openly on the future possibility when some inspiration begins to emerge.[1] Dwelling helps to enhance the achievement of that possibility. In experiential thinking, dwelling or attending on possibilities is a mindfulness-oriented practice that requires discipline, but also the ability to focus without analysis or judgment in place of these processes when one ruminates on a problem. Unfortunately, dwelling and ruminating are viewed by some people as the same thing. The difference in therapy is that ruminating is a reaction to an unresolved mental problem with an obsession toward constantly thinking about it. Whereas, dwelling is taking the time spent needlessly ruminating and giving it intentionality toward positive action of an unresolved mental problem. It is a conscious effort to let one's intuition, unconscious tacit knowledge, and insight emerge on its own, without directly thinking about it (Stanislas 2014).[2] In some cases, it may be one of the goals of experiential therapy is to replace client rumination with dwelling or attending.

The importance of differentiating dwelling from ruminating is that brooding too much on negative events is the biggest predictor of depression and anxiety and determines the level of stress people experience (Cirino 2019). Peoples' psychological response may be a more important factor than what has actually happened to them. For example, what becomes more devastating being raped or thinking about the rape for the next ten years? In my experience in working with victims of rape, the latter seems to do equal damage. Rumination and self-blame have long been accepted by health professionals as part of the problems that can lead to depression and anxiety—the two most common mental health problems (Tartkovsky 2019).

In many ways in therapy, because of intentionality, clients have a choice in the type of thoughts that occupy their thinking that corresponds to their suffering. They can choose ruminating about negative thoughts over and over again, or they can dwell on their thoughts with the intentionality found in thinking with purpose and meaning. In Viktor Frankl's book, *Man's Search for Meaning*, he talks about during his time in Auschwitz how he tried not to ruminate on his condition, but focused his thinking about his wife, and what he was going to do when he saw her again. He said this is what kept him going while in the concentration camps (Frankl 2014). Simply put, rumination over and over again can create loss of purpose and meaning, while intentionally dwelling on something meaningful creates purpose and meaning, and as with Viktor Frankl, sometimes it creates the phenomenon of hope (Frankl 2014). Edmund Husserl was one of a few who understood intentionality. He would say thought is "intentional." It is of the nature of thought to be directed toward or about something (Mabaquiao 2005). Experiential therapists collaborate with the client regarding their thought processes. Are you going to ruminate or are you going to find purpose and meaning in your thinking? Finding purpose and meaning in a client's life is what intentionality is all about in mental health therapy.

Albert Einstein spent years intentionally attending to or dwelling on the theory behind the speed of light and the concept of time. Not by ruminating on this concept, but by attending to it. Letting it find meaning and purpose in his thinking until it intuitively popped out (Moylana, Lombardi, and Moylanc 2016). This may be a strange metaphor to use with the brilliance of Albert Einstein but in effect, Einstein "hatched" the concept of $E = mc$ 2. The thoughts were stored somewhere in his unconscious mind until they eventually came to the surface. He did not ruminate over them, he dwelled on them, not in an analytical way, but in an intuitive way until that "aha moment" brought them to the conscious level of his thinking. Dwelling is more about the purpose connected to intentionality, rather than the purposeless act of ruminating. Dwelling in the sense that at times you are unconsciously creating a comfortable climate and flow where your thinking becomes meaningful to you but not necessarily by laboring over it, but by letting nuanced ideas emerge on their own.

I like to use the word *dwelling* when thinking about intentionality. Intentionality is the realization that we constantly remain unconscious and conscious of something. (Note: I also like the word *attending*, but some people seem to confuse it with ruminating.) Dwelling is one method for accomplishing purpose and meaning in intentionality. This is different than ruminating or worrying. For me, ruminating is thinking in circles while losing one's purpose. Dwelling is based on making a commitment to some purpose except you remain detached from constantly thinking about it, until thoughts emerge that advance your awareness and understanding.

In other words, in therapy, clients make a commitment to understanding their problems, by letting problems go, until new thoughts surface that help give them clarity. They do not try to overthink them. They let thoughts emerge when they are ready. That does not mean that somewhere in their thinking their thoughts have disappeared. The unconscious mind dwells on the commitment to solve a specific problem until the problem is ready to emerge. Metaphorically speaking, much like an aquarium of the unconscious mind filled with personal tacit knowledge such as feelings, thoughts, behaviors, and other unknown phenomena mysteriously connects to moments in the conscious mind, making them meaningful. Again, metaphorically speaking, unlike the explicit knowledge or memories found in the filing cabinets of the hippocampus where your conscious memories are stored. During therapy, they may become less important and valuable than your unconscious tacit knowledge filled with nuances that are emerging on their own.

This client was struggling with the fact that his wife had left him. He was filled with anxiety and depression, and the more he thought about it, the worse he became. The therapist told him that he was ruminating, and that seemed to make matters worse. Finally, the client agreed that he would make a commitment to let his thinking run its course by attending to the divorce, not ruminating on it. The client stopped thinking about his wife but attended to the experience of having a future. He came into the therapist's office the next week and said he had a breakthrough in his divorce experience. Somehow it popped into his head that "gone is gone" and decided that he must move on. So, he went to an old covered bridge, and threw his ring into the river. Whether he did the right thing or not, that was the intentionality that came out of his attending to the thoughts about divorce. Instead of ruminating over why she left, he let the power of attending give him intention and purpose.

This helps to clarify why it is important to give time between therapy sessions, so clients can attend to their problems. I believe that most growth and change does not happen in therapy sessions, but between sessions when clients have the opportunity to, in the privacy of their own minds, attend without judgment or advice. When you are attending to a problem in effect you are letting the problem drift into an unconscious ether of tacit knowledge, not in the act of forgetting about your problem, but by expanding the awareness of a curious mind that is open to whatever happens/happened, allowing the unknown tacit knowledge found in attending, to bring you closer to an awareness of the experience. I cannot tell you how many times I have watched chronic worriers or ruminators become free of the rumination by counterintuitively getting on with their lives through the intentionality found in attending to a problem. Dwelling is based more on trust not control. It is counterintuitive; the more you stop thinking about your problems the more accurate an answer emerges.

This may be the reason that some people say it is important to think with your heart and not with your mind. Dwelling follows different neurological pathways than ruminating (Kounios and Beeman 2016). In therapy, attending is trying to understand a problem through one's instincts, not necessarily one's conscious thoughts. When a client dwells on what was said in therapy, or dwells on understanding their feelings, or dwells on a meaningful future project, goal, or aspirations, he or she is using intuition more than cognition. When a client ruminates, she or he is using cognition over and over again to solve a problem. With dwelling to something in therapy a client can have an insightful "aha" moment, a breakthrough. With ruminating in therapy, a client can overanalyze a problem, and become farther from any possible breakthrough. So, to tell a client/patient to stop thinking about their mental problems is probably the wrong statement to make. First, they most likely have difficulty in stopping an issue that is dominating their thoughts. More accurately it may be to think about your mental problems in a different way. Stop ruminating and start to attend to them.

MINDFULNESS: A FORM OF DWELLING

With the increased popularity of mindfulness, it may be important to point out that mindfulness is experiential, not calculated. It is a method that allows phenomena to emerge. For this reason, both mindfulness and dwelling can be effective together in talk therapy. There is little reason to calculate experiences in mindfulness or dwelling. It is a matter of letting whatever is happening emerge. When clients begin to dwell in therapy, they are experiencing information coming into their senses in real time about the intentionality of the therapy problem under consideration (Singleton 2014). A similar experience happens in mindfulness activities such as meditation, breathing exercises, and so on. Through this commitment to staying in the present and not ruminate about the past or future, mindfulness can help distill mental rumination, help weigh options, tune into a client's intuition, and ultimately make decisions that a client can stand behind.

As a rule, the medical model relies on calculated decisions in most mental health therapy, and in many respects, experienced mental health professionals can be quite accurate in making these decisions. In the world of experience, intuitive decision-making fits more with a non-hypothesis model where decisions can emerge without trying to prove a previous diagnosis. In my experience, it is more common to ruminate over a mental problem that has been labeled from a diagnosis than to attend to a mental problem where the intentionality is to let an answer to the problem emerge. Some of the same experiences happen when using mindfulness techniques in mental health therapy.

At this point, it may be important to point out that not all mindfulness skills come specifically from some form of actual skills training presented on their own such as breathing exercises, meditation, EMDR, or any other mindfulness skills. In mental health therapy, the practice of dwelling in therapy by nonthinking, followed by staying in the present, and eventually returning to the problem through intuition and insight is a form of mindfulness—even though it may not be recognized as a mindful experience.

Another overlooked phenomenon is believing that rumination and dwelling are the same experience. Hopefully, what has been said so far has separated them for both the client and therapist. To the untrained eye, a common response is to believe they are the same, generating statements such as, "Stop thinking about it!" To the trained eye, it may be more accurate to say, "If you are going to focus on your mental problems, try dwelling on them without thinking about them." And, if you again start ruminating, slowly bring your focus back to dwelling, eventually by practicing nonthinking until intuitive information emerges through insight concerning the problem. You are changing constant rumination by the counterintuitive method of attending.[3]

CASE STUDY

Linda was a young woman in her thirties who struggled with gaining forty pounds in the past year. This was accompanied by having chest pains and anxiety attacks. What was unusual about the panic attacks is they happened every night around seven o'clock. She was concerned about her physical health but also her feelings concerning relationships with men. Over a year ago, she went through a painful breakup with an abusive boyfriend, and since that time her personal view of herself had changed for the worse. Linda was not a person who let herself slide into negativity, so her current behavior was puzzling her. She had to figure out what was going on, so she would constantly ruminate over her problems only to have more anxiety and more pain at this unusual 7 o'clock hour.

She had been to a medical model mental health therapist who referred her to a psychiatrist where she received the antianxiety medication, Ativan. She was told to take the medicine when these attacks began, and that strategy numbed the anxiety but did little to address the pains in her chest. The drug prescription was followed by a diagnosis of general anxiety disorder with obsessive-compulsive tendencies. The obsessive-compulsive part was attributed to her constant rumination over her psychological problems, since her chest pains through tests eliminated them as a physical problem. She was now overweight, but outside of that, she was normal. For someone who used to be dynamic, assertive, and successful, the answers given to her by the psychiatrist were unacceptable. She did not see herself as an anxious person, and her chest pains remained a mystery except professionals telling her that the pain was a symptom of anxiety.

In desperation, she contacted a friend who knew a friend who knew about a mental health therapist who had a reputation for listening more than judging. She got an appointment to see Kyle, a middle-aged, compassionate woman who greeted her in her office. Linda sat down for an engaging hour-and-a-half discussion about how Linda saw herself gaining weight, the past abusive relationship, the confusing chest pains, and rumination over what to do about them. She told Kyle that the medication was helpful, but the diagnosis was not. She explained how she was noted for solving her problems but in this case, she was going in circles which seemed to make things worse.

The message that Kyle conveyed to Linda made sense. First, she described anxiety as being counterintuitive: the harder you try to solve something the worse it can get. Linda immediately saw this happening with herself. Second, Kyle pointed out that the trauma caused by an abusive boyfriend can trigger other traumas in life, making the combination of traumas overwhelming. Third, the gaining weight and how she saw herself seemed to be at odds. "You have basically told me the weight gain is not you." Kyle finally said that what she was pointing out are not the words of an expert, but someone who has watched other dynamic women struggle with these issues. I am speaking to you from the experiences of others, but there may be something to gain from their wisdom.

Linda left Kyle's office with the sense of having a meaningful conversation with someone, not someone who was trying to diagnose and label her, but a person who seemed curious enough to engage her with respect and intelligence. For whatever reasons, this meant a lot to Linda. She felt that she had someone on her side, not someone who was going to fix her. The following sessions proved her observation to be true. They discussed the trauma she felt from the previous relationship with the abusive boyfriend, and just the venting alone helped Linda feel more normal when thinking about relationships in general. She admitted that adding the extra weight was affecting her self-esteem, but diet and exercise did not seem to work at this time. More importantly she prided herself in being an intelligent person, but she was confused about her chest pains and her inability to figure out where they were coming from.

Linda reminded her of the counterintuitive nature of anxiety, and how her attempts to solve the problem with her chest pains was causing her to ruminate and go in circles, even though with dynamic people it seems the most obvious thing to do. They both agreed that the chest pains were trying to tell her something but ruminating over what was wrong with her had little positive effect. She also told Linda that most of her clients who successfully change do not ruminate, but continue to attend to either what was said in therapy, or keep their problems in mind during other moments of their day. She used the metaphor that if therapy was a play, she was not the actor or the director in the play. She explained to Linda, that it was her job because she had the right to act out her life as she saw fit, and she also had the right to direct the course her life would take. Kyle explained that her job was that of a stagehand. She was responsible for setting the stage so acting and directing can happen.

Kyle said that to set the stage properly, there is one thing that may need to change. Linda, you have admitted that ruminating over your chest pains has not worked. How about if we give those chest pains a purpose and a different meaning for what they secretly are hiding from us. I am suggesting, in my experience, how awareness of a problem and changing a problem is more of an intuitive process, or if you like the word, mindfulness process. How about if we consider giving your chest pains some positive meaning? Instead of ruminating over how to get rid of the pain, how about dedicating some important meaningful activity as an alternative to ruminating over how to fix the pain. Kyle also told Linda that she normally does not give homework assignments, but instead of her trying to explain what she meant as an expert, read the book by Viktor Frankl, *Man's Search for Meaning*. He spent time in the concentration camp at Auschwitz, and instead of ruminating over his pain, he attended to a vision of his wife and their time together after the war. He said that attending to something positive saved him from his own despair.

Linda's plan was not created by Kyle. Her answer was around seven o'clock when the pain began, she dedicated the pain to exercising on her cross-trainer until she was physically tired. However, just physical exercise was not enough. The intentionality of her action also had to be established. Her dedication to the pain was her way of attending to the pain through exercise. The pain took on a more positive meaning for her. She was not going to figure it out. She was going to let the awareness of the pain emerge through exercise. Linda began to lose weight. Her anxiety levels dropped. And, during one crucial exercise period an epiphany came to her.

When she met with Kyle, purpose and meaning filled the room. She told her that when she was seven years old her uncle sexually abused her and not surprising, it was at seven o'clock at night. Kyle said that sometimes when we try to hide from our pain our bodies are smarter than our minds. It sounds like your body had enough of hiding and was trying to tell you something. When you started to attend to your accumulated trauma, your body must have felt you learned something, and no more hiding was necessary. Kyle said, "I know my explanation is more of a metaphor, and is not scientifically grounded in research, but it is the best I can do." Linda said, "Well, it sounds good to me. It is not that important as to how it is understood. What is more important is to feel as though I am moving on." The rest of their therapy together was reinforcing and establishing plans for the future, and to remember that sometimes it is better to attend to problems rather than ruminate over them.

DISCUSSION

In the case study, it appeared more important for Linda to work through her experiences with abuse, chest pains, and anxiety than being diagnosed as someone who had these symptoms. What may be sufficient for the mental health professional may not be as sufficient for the client. Surprisingly, in the case study, both models were accurate, one from a diagnostic viewpoint, the other from an experiential point of view. In mental health therapy, the empirical viewpoint has prevailed, over the regrets of such icons as Sigmund Freud, Carl Rogers, and Viktor Frankl. Dwelling is one example of a phenomenon that seems lost within the scientifically focused medical model, even though it has a long history of being effective in human relations from Buddhism to mindfulness training.

The intentionality found in experiential thinking can give rise to attending as a major part of mental health therapy. As portrayed in the case study, even suffering can find meaning if we choose it. Clients have found deep meaning in Viktor Frankl's formula for meaning. He states that "Suffering - Meaning = Despair" (Frankl 2014). In the case study, when Linda put meaning to her suffering, she "dodged the bullet" of suffering without meaning. Her intentionality is in restoring a positive life, not ruminating over how to eliminate her pain. She figured a way to work through her pain, not by covering it up with psychotropic drugs or diagnostic explanations.

Neuroscience has taught us that we can have only one dominating thought at a time, even though we have thousands of thoughts each day. By ruminating on our thoughts, we run the risk of thinking the same dominating thoughts over and over again (Derhaine 2019). This does not take away the uncertainty found in anxiety but adds to it. Dwelling also does not stop us from thinking about the uncertainty found in anxiety but channels it into some form of non-thinking while attending closely to the problem at hand. It becomes proactive not reactive. It avoids learned helplessness regarding our thoughts when ruminating. Dwelling helps in the creation of resilience and grit by working through anxiety and pain. We become more involved with our own recovery.

One obvious question may be, "Does that mean the medical model of mental health is not effective?" To answer such a question, it must be preceded with a choice of answers. If what you want is to reduce the symptoms of a mental health disorder, a medical model of therapy has proven to be effective for some people. If what you want is to work through painful experiences where some are classified as disorders, a more experiential approach has proven effective for some people. In the case study, Linda did find relief from anxiety and pain by using the medical model. If all that she wanted out of a medical model was Ativan, and believing she had general anxiety disorder with secondary symptoms of obsessive-compulsive disorder, the therapy would have been satisfactory.

Linda was working from a more curious mind and was not satisfied with only information and analysis from an expert about her problems. She wanted to tell her story and have someone listen. She was looking for a therapist who could engage her in a dialogue about certain experiences in her life. She was not looking for a skilled person to fix her life. She wanted to understand more clearly what had happened to her over the past number of years, and what she could do about it. For those seeking therapy, it may come down to perspective. The medical model has its own perspective on what is normal or abnormal but with no real guidelines to what proves to be normality (Hansen 2016). The experiential model moves away from who is normal or abnormal and focuses more on a holistic approach that not only includes behavior, thoughts, and feelings but also includes neuroscience and environment. Here is where the richness of client stories in therapy can be told from many different angles, and not rely only on the angle owned in therapy by the scientific method.

Acceptance and Commitment Therapy

For those experiential therapists who want a format for teaching "dwelling" outside of therapy or inside it when appropriate, acceptance and commitment therapy (ACT) takes all the elements of attending but in a more structured format (Hayes 2005). (Quite frankly, I do not know why ACT is given its roots in CBT when it obviously, to me, has a strong connection to existential/phenomenological thinking.) ACT can be used to teach clients attending skills to deal with painful thoughts and feelings. Clients can learn to clarify what is truly important and meaningful in their thinking. It is one of the more effective methods to counteract rumination in a client's negative experiences.

Rogers and Dwelling

As someone who has taught graduate mental health counseling students for over thirty years, it has become clear to me the importance of using the skill of attending (dwelling) not only by the therapist but also by the client. Carl Rogers in the early part of the 1950s pointed out certain conditions for a healthy therapeutic climate in therapy including positive regard, empathy, and genuineness (Rogers 2003). These skills take the therapist away from the role of expert and place she or he in the position of being one's authentic self. Students are taught to attend by bracketing their thoughts and feelings and focus on whatever the client finds meaningful in the experience between therapist and client. When clients ruminate over their mental problems, they put themselves in the role of expert, believing they have the expertise to solve these problems. Metaphorically speaking, "It may be hard to see the picture when you are inside the frame." One's responsibility as mental health therapists may be to help clients secure their position as human beings. Part of the client's predicament may be trying to practice an expertise instead of attending to mental problems as a part of the human experience.

In the case study, we see Kyle help Linda to attend rather than ruminate over her mental problems. She clears the air for Linda to practice the intentionality behind nonthinking by creating a structure for purpose and meaning to exist. Part of the brilliance demonstrated by Carl Roger was his stance away from practicing an expertise and in its place attending closely to the experience of the client. Many of the factors in previous chapters are enhanced by both client and therapist practicing the art of attending. For example, momentum can increase, dialogue becomes richer, nuances gain more importance, and wisdom begins to replace knowledge.

These are not skills emanating from our scientific discoveries in mental health, but skills indicative of human experience. It is one of natural history's greatest gifts, the ability of humans to attend to the world around them, instead of following an inflexible pattern in science. It is what saves us from the inability to make adjustments in our everyday world. A pattern of rumination does the opposite by thinking we can overcome mental problems by worrying about them, rather than allowing them to run their course. It is better to let anxiety run its course when experiencing it, than trying to think our way out of it. No one wants to extend such an experience as anxiety by ruminating over what can be done to end it and find themselves in an anxiety loop causing more anxiety.

A Beatles's song keeps coming to me when trying to describe attending, even though I know this song has become a bit of a cliché. "When I find myself in times of trouble Mother Mary comes to me. Speaking words of wisdom, let it be." Unfortunately, rumination does the opposite of letting it be, or letting it turn productive. I believe we all need moments in time to let awareness of negative experiences turn productive. The skill of dwelling gives us that time. Not everything can be figured out by cognitively analyzing what has happened to us. Sometimes we need to trust the process that nonthinking brings to resolving problems. Experiential thinkers describe dwelling as a disciplined naivete. The therapist clears their mind of all assumptions about the client, but in a disciplined way where the intentionality of the therapist's commitment, structures, and purpose gain meaning in therapy. It seems common sense would tell us the clients can do the same.

NOTES

1. "I think 99 times and find nothing. I stop thinking, swim in silence, and the truth comes to me." Albert Einstein. 2013. *The Ultimate Quotable Einstein*. Princeton, NJ: Princeton University Press. Attending or dwelling fits closely with the attitudes and beliefs of such figures as Albert Einstein. His understanding of intuition and insight made him explore wisdom and imagination over knowledge.

2. Such is the case for those experiential therapists who allow themselves to attend or dwell on a future project or person. "I never made one of my discoveries through

the process of rational thinking." Albert Einstein. 2013. *The Ultimate Quotable Einstein*. Princeton, NJ: Princeton University Press. The dwelling (attending) process in therapy finds itself ahead of rational thinking when the patterns of a client's experiences surpass the client or the therapist with their clarity.

3. Dwelling is not primarily inhabiting but taking care of and creating that space within which something comes into its own and flourishes. Martin Heidegger. 2019. *Being and Time*. Eastford, CT: Martino Fine Books.

Chapter 12

Working through Suffering versus Relieving All Suffering

The medical model goal is to relieve all suffering connected to an illness (Egnew 2009). That is one reason why the mental health medical model uses psychotropic drugs, and other forms of therapy techniques. They believe by taking away symptoms it will also take away suffering. This thinking follows in the footsteps of physical medicine where an expert does not want to cure half a disease, but all of it. Except, for example, surgeons do not have to contend with outside personal experiences when operating on patients. Medical model mental health therapists who focus on the outside might consider adding the patient's experiences when relieving suffering. Yet, some of these professionals in the field of mental health believe the role as a mental health provider is to eliminate suffering within the boundaries of symptoms connected to their treatment plans.

The phenomenological and trauma-informed care therapists are more concerned with the human experience of working through suffering, not only eliminating suffering connected to symptoms but also other human experiences. The idea is based on the assumption that some clients can become more resilient and can help normalize their suffering by working through their personal experiences that caused suffering. When eliminating suffering in a medical model of mental health, it is because suffering is considered unnecessary. In actual practice, we are perhaps more helpful as professionals when we assist clients in choosing what is necessary and unnecessary suffering. Through the freedom of choice, clients can begin to eliminate unnecessary suffering, and work through their necessary suffering (Hansen 2017). The experiential thinker believes clients can make a choice to experience their suffering and get relief, or directly face suffering themselves, or to face suffering when they are ready, and this is where confusion can erupt around the healing process regarding suffering.

Do clients know when their suffering is necessary and when it is not? Very little confusion is connected with physical suffering. For the most part, a person experiencing physical suffering will come to the conclusion that it is unnecessary. The same conclusion impulsively can be applied to emotional suffering.

Take, for example, that unnecessary suffering can be numbed out through drug and alcohol addiction. In the short term, that assumption is true. One can be as successful, at first, by numbing emotional suffering as opposed to facing it. Unfortunately, emotional suffering may re-traumatize a person after the numbing wares off. Technically speaking there is not much difference when human beings physically or emotionally begin to heal from their suffering. The actual healing process may seem very different, but both in physical and emotional healing the people can feel worse before they feel better.

In physical healing, a person cuts his hand. The hand is immediately filled with pain. Yet, when the hand begins to heal, there is a period where suffering may become more intense then when it was originally cut. The difference is the person can visualize the changes taking place in the healing of the cut. It may throb, have sharp painful moments, and possibly unimaginable irritation. Even though it may present symptoms beyond the level of pain caused by the original cut, the person can see the difference, and can accept suffering as part of the normal healing process (Ladd 2016).

Emotional pain is similar to physical pain except for one important difference. If a client is experiencing deep emotional pain in life, it may be hard to convince the client who is now healing that it is actually taking place. Even though they may experience emotional healing that is causing as much pain as physical healing, people may have trouble visualizing it. This is one of the dilemmas of being a mental health therapist. How do you convince clients that emotional pain is beginning to heal, when they experience equal amounts of suffering when going through the healing process? The experience between client and therapist during healing may be just as painful as the original suffering, with no visual way of determining whether healing is taking place. A client's perception may be that the pain is getting worse and the therapist is ineffective.

One of the assumptions made about emotional wounds in mental health therapy is quite different than assumptions made about physical wounds. With physical wounds, the healing process is visible to the wounded person and to others involved in the healing process. Emotional wounds are not that easy to visualize, especially when clients have gone out of their way to hide them from their experience.

In mental health therapy, some clients who start to heal from their original pain, question whether they are getting worse, and believe they are living their suffering all over again. There can be no visualized acknowledgment that anything is getting better because the suffering may actually *feel* worse. If a client cannot visualize the healing process, some make the assumption that the suffering *is getting* worse. This phenomenon also applies to those friends and relatives surrounding the client. If the client has an episode of acute emotional suffering, friends and relatives might also assume they are going back to the original suffering which can have a negative influence on client healing.

In a medical model form of therapy, the reality is simply that the above awareness may seldom take place. From the belief that all suffering pertaining to symptom reduction must be eliminated, psychotropic drugs have fulfilled that mandate in a most ubiquitous manner. Patients may descend into a condition referred to as learned helplessness where the expert knows best. Where patients passively wait for the drug or drugs to kick in to relieve their suffering. Patients can become reliant on Big Pharma to relieve their physical, as well as their emotional suffering, without a thought of the possibility of working through it. Experiential therapists struggle with this reality, especially when they believe that working through some forms of suffering may be necessary for client growth and change. The quick fix of the medical model of mental health therapy is hard to dispute in a culture that expects suffering to be quickly taken away. Ironically, physical and emotional healing follow similar responses, euphemistically and possibly accurately described as, "No Pain No Gain"—at least from a phenomenological/existential perspective.

However, there is a difference between pain and suffering, and this applies to emotional and physical pain. When wounded, pain is inevitable, suffering is not. It depends on one's attitude toward pain. According to one's attitude, emotional and physical pain can be modified, according to how much someone decides to suffer. In an experiential model, approaching a client's emotional suffering, and determining what suffering is necessary, remains a high priority. As in grieving the death of a loved one, an experiential perspective would regard grieving as necessary suffering, based on it being a natural and healthy phenomenon in one's experience. Regarding unnecessary suffering, a client may be so much in pain that the ability to speak about the trauma has become impossible. The experiential therapist might spend time helping the client understand their pain and the suffering that goes with it, or they may refer the client to a psychiatrist to obtain psychotropic drugs to eliminate this unnecessary part of pain and suffering. The discriminating awareness of the experiential therapist does not deny the value in eliminating some forms of pain and suffering. However, necessary suffering can become paramount by working through one's emotional problems, in order to find meaning in one's life—to obtain resilience, regain confidence, to place the locus of control back into the soul of the client (Rogers 2003).

There is noticeably a difference in philosophy regarding suffering found in the mental health medical model, as compared to the experiential model. With contemporary culture, quick fixes and a belief that pain and suffering connected to symptoms must be eliminated challenge a model grounded in human experience, not to mention human suffering. In response, one only has to recognize the power contained in human interaction to answer this question. Not only is the *therapeutic alliance* proven as one of the most effective phenomena in the field of mental health, but it also is based on the experience of trust between therapist and client (Safran et al. 2014). With this alliance, the experiential therapist can describe the difference between necessary and unnecessary suffering. The development of a therapeutic alliance also refers to trust between two human beings. The therapist can ask the client to bond together in working through necessary suffering, while at the same time, make sure there are remedies in place to eliminate the pain involved in unnecessary suffering. This is why one of my contentions is that trust is more powerful than control in mental health therapy.

The experiential therapist does not claim to have the answers of how to control all suffering but asks the client to trust in human interaction between them, to separate meaningful suffering that may be a part of their human experiences from suffering that is unnecessary, that negatively impacts their experiences. It is more of an existential perspective that suffering is a part of human existence and cannot be judged simply as unacceptable within the experiences of clients. That is not to say this form of therapy welcomes suffering, but it does speak to the reality that it exists and needs to be carefully understood both positively and negatively.

I have made a point in the beginning of therapy with some very anxious clients, to let my view of pain and suffering be understood. Not in the sense that clients will have to suffer to complete therapy, but in the difference between necessary and unnecessary suffering. I comment on how together we will approach both, if or when suffering becomes a part of the therapy process. Or, if a client is already in pain, how do we determine whether it is necessary or unnecessary. Being honest about pain and suffering has worked for me, especially with clients demonstrating high anxiety. It allows clients to know they are a part of confronting the reality that suffering is in both of our hands. Furthermore, they may have the opportunity to trust relieving suffering and not remain under the control of an expert, who intends to get rid of pain and suffering connected to symptoms.

Second, I have shied away from explaining both forms of suffering from a scholarly perspective. The less scientific use of metaphors seems fitting within the realm of an experiential therapist. The metaphor that "a scar is not a wound" has worked for me in making clients aware of the similarities and differences between physical healing and emotional healing. First, an explanation that healing both physical and emotional follow a similar process. This leads to the difference and ease in recognizing physical healing, where it becomes more difficult in recognizing emotional healing. When you have a physical wound that is healing, you are eventually left with a scar that on occasions may flare up for any number of reasons—weather, stress, and so on. There is no mention of the scar tragically turning back into a wound (Ladd 2016). However, when you have an emotional wound that is healing, it becomes more difficult to eventually recognize it as a scar. Assumptions can be made during therapy that the former wound has opened up and the full extent of pain and suffering will begin all over again. Experiential therapists may describe how healing can be misunderstood when working with clients, who present patterns of anxiety, or depression, or other patterns with uncertain outcomes. Where moments during the healing process signal defeat and a return the severity of the original emotional wound. It may be that therapists have an obligation to describe the healing process both physical and emotional, and how suffering enters into that process.

This may be why some clients rather numb their pain and suffering rather than face it. It is popular because numbing works. Ask any alcoholic or drug addict whether this is true. They might tell you that it does not take it away, but it does work temporarily, and this is a choice that clients make when coping with emotional pain and suffering. The question raised is whether clients are satisfied with coping with their suffering, or do they want to overcome it, even though what remains might be a scar to remind them of their achievement. The previous statement is not a vendetta against the medical model of therapy or Big Pharma. With some disorders such as bipolar, schizophrenia, and other disorders the use of psychotropic drugs may be mandatory in relieving unnecessary suffering. However, with these disorders the experience of embarrassment, inferiority, alienation, and inhumane treatment may require a journey through the necessary suffering connected to human growth and personal identity.

CASE STUDY

Jake was a Vietnam veteran who had survived thirty years of suffering after the war where some of his fellow soldiers did not make it. Even though he had developed into an experienced contractor, his drug and alcohol problems persisted during this time period. For some time, he had been diagnosed with chronic depression and was taking Lexapro, an antidepressant drug. The symptoms of depression were helped by the drug, but his ongoing bouts with feeling depressed would still flare up at any moment during the year. This reality caused him to ruminate about "when the next shoe would drop" causing increased experiences of anxiety. Overall, he seemed to suffer from what medical model experts would call dysthymia or mild depression. However, the diagnosis did not seem to change because the drugs also worked in taking away some of the depression connected to his experiences.

Finally, Jake's wife, Jean, talked him into seeing a more experiential therapist, who focused more on talking than on medicine. The suggestion was made regarding Jake wanting to bring up thoughts of Vietnam, even though past experiences in his world were long gone, at least according to Jean. Jake entered Emma's counseling office with skepticism written all over his face. "What could a young, female therapist understand about my traumatic experiences from the Vietnam War?" The first thing that Jake learned was that Emma was more interested in listening than in talking, as Jake tried to figure out how this young therapist could help him. When Jake returned home after therapy, Jean asked, "How did it go?" Jake replied, "I really don't know but I feel better. She is a nice young girl who seemed interested in my life and did not probe me for information." Jean responded, "I have been telling you for years it was important to talk with someone other than family." Jake responded that she said something about that. She said, "It is hard to see the picture when you are inside the frame." Jake said, "I guess that gets you off the hook about listening to my war stories."

Emma made a point that it was important to vent his stories of the war, and that Jake seemed relieved after voicing them. She also said that it seemed odd that between the medication and the venting the stories still were the predominate topic of discussion in the five weeks they had been seeing each other. Emma believed that sadness was an important phenomenon to work through, and she admitted that some people take years to work through their sadness. She hoped the venting was helping him work through his sadness, and she believed from her perspective that it seemed helpful.

However, Emma was intuitively picking up that something was being held back, and took the risk to ask the question: "Is there anything you feel you cannot tell me about Vietnam?" Jake looked down in tears. He faced her with a guilt-ridden glance and said, "Yes, but I am ashamed to mention it, even to Jean." Emma replied, "When you are ready, consider mentioning it to me." Jake became silent and chose not to talk much until the session was over. Emma did not press the issue but joined in on talking about their families and how attached they were to them.

That week, Jake struggled with disturbing thoughts to the point that his rumination began overwhelming him. At his appointment with Emma, he commented that what he was about to say might be more painful than anything he had divulged in his life. Emma commented, "Sounds like you are ready to gain courage to start the healing whatever it is that has been bothering you. Sometimes, we do not emotionally understand our healing because it seems too painful, but it may be healing just the same."

Jake began by telling Emma that he was in a heavy equipment unit in the army, and that his job was to drive a large crane for building temporary bridges across bodies of water. One day his commanding officer asked him to drive a wounded soldier to an army hospital, a significant distance from where he was working. Jake said that "it may have been that I did not have the time to think, or I took the easy way out by choosing a friend to take his place on the crane." His friend only lived about forty-five minutes from his home in the United States. Jake continued, "While driving the wounded soldier, his friend was killed on the crane from a round of mortar fire, and he never recovered from the incident. Emma said, "Jake it sounds like this incident is different than the others. You expressed sadness when telling those stories, but I get the feeling that we are now talking about guilt." Jake said, "Yes, guilt and shame." Jake continued, "A few days before the incident my friend had shared a picture of his newborn child, and how happy he was to be a father, and within one day, all his dreams had ended because of me." Emma sat quietly and did not try to rationalize such ineffective answers such as "it was not your fault" or "you cannot control what happens in life." She knew those expert statements were not appropriate, and it was Jake's time of reflection, and she chose to listen and remain quiet.

The week passed and Jake again sat down with Emma and asked her, "What do you think I should do?" Emma responded, "Well, Jake here is what we know. Guilt has replaced sadness in your mind with this one incident. You have a connection to your friend, but you also have a connection to his family. You have spent thirty-five years burying this story at great expense to you going through unnecessary suffering. You admit that the medication has worked in helping with other stories, but not with this one." This put Jake in a difficult situation because he had no answers to the accuracy of Emma's comments. Emma had set the stage for Jake to have choices, without making a decision, and without approaching his choices as an expert.

Next week, Jake entered Emma's office with fear on his face. He said, "Emma, I know what I have to do; even though, I am scared that it could be bringing back the pain and suffering from the past. I have to call my friend's family and talk to them, and also visit the grave of my friend and say my statement to him." Emma replied that she would support his choice, and that it showed great courage to work through a painful memory from the past.

That night Jake called the number he had looked up, and on the other end of the phone a deep-throated voice responded to Jakes request to talk with his friend's wife. The person on the other end said that she was not there but he was her son. Jake shared his reason for calling, and his friend's son was overjoyed that he wanted to contact his mother. As it turned out, his friend's son was in the marine corps and was visiting his mother, just by chance, and told Jake to call back tomorrow.

The day came and the wife of Jake's friend answered the phone call. She was also elated about him making contact with her and invited him and his wife to visit. Jake came back to therapy and told Emma the whole story. She was highly supportive and encouraged him to make the visit.

According to Jake, these were some of the scariest moments in his life, far beyond Vietnam when he pulled up to the door of his fallen friend's house. When the door opened, a small, fragile woman and a six-foot five-inch male with smiles and tears on their faces met with Jake, who also had tears streaming down his face. It was one of those nuances in experience that will be remembered for a lifetime. What Jake discovered was that he had intimate information to share with his friend's family, and that they were eager to hear it. He also expressed how guilty he felt, and he wished it would have been him. They graciously heard him out, but frankly wanted information on their loved one. For a number of hours, he shared his experience that he and his friend encountered in Vietnam. Near the end of the conversation, the large marine asked if on another occasion whether he would accompany them to his grave. Jake was a bit in shock, but Jean accepted for both of them.

At the grave site both families allowed Jake to say his statement to his long-lost friend. With tears in his eyes, he shared any number of things that until this day, he could not fully remember what he said, and that is what he said to Emma at his next visit. She told Jake that what he said at the grave site may or may not come back with time, but the important point is he suffered through the experience until reaching the other side of his reconciliation with his friend, and with himself. It turned out to be the necessary thing to do. Now he can feel sad about those days in Vietnam because many of them are sad, but his guilt about his friend is disappearing, and in its place is an important part of growth and change in his life.

DISCUSSION

Viktor Frankl in searching for meaning reiterates in numerous writings that, at times, it is necessary to experience the pain and suffering that comes with life's traumas. Some of this suffering is necessary while at other times, it is not (Frankl 2009). In the case study, Jake experienced unnecessary suffering in recalling the traumatic memories of Vietnam. Through medication and venting with the therapist, Emma, he made attempts to work through his unnecessary suffering. However, with one meaningful experience in his life, Jake decided that getting closure on his guilt and shame was necessary suffering when meeting with his friend's family and making peace by visiting his friend's grave.

For those who practice mindfulness, suffering may be a meaningful experience in life and should not be avoided (Coleman 2019). The avoidance of suffering may lead to further suffering. One can see the countless amount of time Jake put into avoiding the one major trauma in his life that acted as a filter for other life experiences, for over thirty years. So, there are arguments suggesting suffering can be beneficial or warranted, but much is unnecessary, and self-created (Coleman 2019). Jake's shame created unnecessary suffering even though he initially believed he was facing his suffering through medication. The intuitive power of experiential therapists in noticing important nuances in the dialogue between therapist and client may be more effective than the therapist spending time looking for symptoms that match the client's diagnosis and devising solutions to eliminate these symptoms. Intuitively, Emma noticed that Jake may be avoiding trauma in his life that spoke to a more negative experience that he was avoiding, all leading Jake to his eventual necessary suffering.

The medical model of therapy places suffering in a secondary role to client symptoms connected to a disorder. From experiential thinking, pain and suffering become a major concern in life experiences and may be viewed as a more vital concern than client symptoms. In the case study, the medical model of therapy relied on medication to reduce Jake's symptoms of depression; even though, his depression was symptomatic of his avoidance of necessary suffering. Until he faced and worked through the necessary suffering of guilt and shame caused by feeling responsible for losing a friend, he may need medical model solutions for the rest of his life. Conversely, Emma helped Jake put meaning to his suffering, where he now was empowered to become a meaning maker in his life experiences, when he visited his friend's family and together grieving the loss of a loved one (Voros 2016). It may be that experiential therapists need to recognize and address the pain and suffering of their clients and make suffering that seems meaningless become meaningful (Miller and Rollnik 2012).

Viktor Frankl in his book, *Man's Search for Meaning*, describes how the only thing that the Nazis were unable to take away was his choice as to how to respond to suffering. This may make it important to show the difference between pain and suffering. Pain is biologically based on a stimulus/response phenomenon. For example, the stimulus may be some traumatic experience that hits you, whether physical or emotional, and the response is pain. In one's life, the experience of pain is inevitable. However, suffering is different. It may be why experiential therapists want to create awareness of the difference between necessary and unnecessary suffering. When faced with suffering, a person can choose to make a space, a brief moment of reflection, between stimulus and response, and through this space make a choice between necessary and unnecessary suffering. The medical model of therapy normally does not recognize the choice between necessary and unnecessary suffering. In my estimation it puts an overreliance on the stimulus/response phenomenon of pain. Under these conditions all suffering is unnecessary. The stimulus/response experience is more directed toward treating the pain not the suffering.

Patients take psychotropic drugs in mental health therapy to rid themselves of the pain that accompanies their disorders. Attached to eliminating the pain is the hope of eliminating the suffering attached to the pain. An experiential therapist sees pain and suffering as two different phenomena. It is understandable that as found in a medical model of therapy that eliminating pain can be beneficial to client symptoms reduction. Yet, regarding suffering, awareness of necessary and unnecessary suffering is the choice to reduce it, or work through it. Jake in the case study chose both; he realized two methods for reducing unnecessary suffering were to take psychotropic drugs and to vent with his therapist about painful experiences that he wanted to let go while in therapy. On the other hand, he also realized that one specific experience needed to be worked through, in order to find future meaning in his life. As Viktor Frankl might say, "One's ability to retain that degree of psycho-spiritual autonomy in the most horrific circumstances imaginable provides a remarkable example of intra-personal strength, grace under extreme duress, and the power of personal choice" (Frankl 1973).[1] Pain is unavoidable. Suffering is not. Suffering occurs in response to thoughts such as "why me?!", "it isn't fair!", "this is horrible!", "I can't stand it!" It may be that avoiding necessary suffering can lead to an increase in unnecessary suffering. For thirty years in the case study, Jake avoided the importance of necessary suffering with the death of his friend in Vietnam. One can speculate how much impact that had on experiencing unnecessary suffering, not to mention his bouts with depression. The meaning that comes out of suffering for the experiential therapist may be why the focus is more on experience than on symptoms emanating from the DSM. As far as personal experience, for the medical model therapist, symptoms have more meaning for therapist in backing up a diagnosis found in the DSM. However, for clients understanding the difference between pain and suffering may be the turning point in therapy where clients decide how to rid themselves of unnecessary pain and suffering, and how to use necessary suffering to gain resilience, perspective, and confidences in future experiences.

Even pain takes on a different perspective when being aware of the phenomenon of suffering. As demonstrated in pain emanating from a physical injury, the suffering in healing seems necessary and acceptable. If the therapist can make clients aware of the meaning behind an emotional injury to the point of being acceptable, who can speculate how many psychological disorders would be cast into a different light, where changing one's experiential choices regarding suffering has an impact on one's mental disorders. Neurologically, positive thoughts lead to positive emotions and behavior, while the opposite is correct for negative thinking. Awareness of the impact suffering has on the human condition opens that space between stimulus and response, where inevitable pain can be a choice as to how one decides to suffer or not suffer. For the experiential therapist, having choices is one of the first elements contained in emotional freedom. In the case study, Jake made the choice to work through necessary suffering, and for Jake it was the right thing to do.

NOTE

1. I had the privilege of working with Viktor Frankl in the late seventies as his graduate assistant, and it was a lesson in the difference between pain and suffering. Being a newly baptized Vietnam War veteran, Frankl took me under his wing while doing my doctoral dissertation on *Resentment of Authority: A Phenomenological Approach*. San Diego, CA: U.S. International University, 1976. From the pain I was experiencing, he showed me how to put meaning to pain. I realized that it was a choice to suffer or to not suffer. One of the major shifts in my life experiences was to welcome the wisdom found in necessary suffering.

Chapter 13

Neuroscience and Human Experience versus Neuroscience and the Medical Model

NEUROSCIENCE AND MEDICAL MODEL THINKING

The irony in diagnosing for mental illness from a medical model is that it has little do with neuroscience. In forming the DSM, a group of professionals in mental health, mostly psychiatrists, got together and formed committees to observe behaviors in their practices, and combine these observations through a collection of samples from many similar professionals, along with feedback from patients about their symptoms. They agreed through statistical probability on a cluster of symptoms indicative of specific behaviors. They designated time lines for their severity, and finally gave them labels. Nowhere in that process is neuroscience called upon to help capture the designated disorders being evaluated. Even though advances in neuroscience have exploded, mental health shows little progress neurologically toward improved clinical procedures for patients with mental problems. The gap between neuroscience and clinical procedures could be classified as mindless neuroscience versus brainless psychiatry (Insel and Cuthbert 2015).[1]

The use of psychotropic drugs as the backbone of the medical model's credibility and practice has shifted in the field of neuroscience. Regarding treatment, the psychopharmacology industry has researched, and has made strong inroads into the chemical makeup of our brains. In spite of this, psychopharmacology may have leveled off in the field of neuroscience. The new direction grounded in the idea is that we can better understand complex human emotion and behavior by understanding neural networks (Duerstewtiz, Koppe, and Meyers-Lindenberg 2019). A new wave of interest is beginning to rise within neuroscience. The surge of activity is not with the concepts that gave rise to psychotropic drugs, but in the extent to which research and treatment are being driven by a desire to identify and modify key brain circuits (Wasserman and Wasserman 2019). The starkest indication that drugs are increasingly being thought of as yesterday's cutting edge comes from the little-mentioned fact that almost all the major drug companies have closed, or curtailed their drug discovery programs for mental and neurological disorders (Bell 2013). The realization for these companies is that little in the way of genuine innovation has taken place since the major classes of psychiatric drugs were discovered in the 1950s (Ghanem 2014). New drugs have regularly appeared since then, often with fewer side effects, but most are little better in terms of effectiveness (Baumeister 2016).

Adding to this shift in focus, combining neuroscience with medical model diagnosis has not been productive, where little transferrable research is available to this point in time. The current model of mental health diagnosis in use since the days of creating the DSM is solely on observation by clinicians, and the reporting of symptoms by patients. Right now, in psychiatry we don't think about the brain at all when we are making a diagnosis or planning a treatment (White 2016).

This does not mean that neuroscience is not on the verge of generating progress. Beginning with neural imaging techniques, to noninvasive electrical brain stimulation, to selective activation of neurons using laser light for research, the field of neuroscience has erupted, yet little has resulted in improvements in caring for patients with mental illness (Underwood 2019). In the future, neuroscience is looking for a concept of the brain that can match research in psychiatry that includes combining a DSM form of diagnosis with the circuitry, networks, and electrical communication found dynamically in the brain. The circuits, networks, approach focuses on how the billions of neurons in the brain communicate with one another via electrical signals. It cuts across the current broad diagnostic categories like anxiety or depression, with the hope of creating a new understanding of how mental illness works neurologically (Abbott 2019).

Yet, connecting neuroscience to the statistical methods used to form the DSM may be just one alternative, and not one based on a more personal and experiential form of mental health diagnosis. In 2020, the DSM 5 has not been successful in balancing diagnosis and treatment with neuroscience. However, years ago, phenomenology (the study of experience) explained why "the talking cure" changes one's neurological functioning. This has been argued ever since Heidegger's and Merleau-Ponty's work in the first half of the last century (Adams 2020). Phenomenology shows the brain to be a system within the broader system of a person's being-in-the-world, and a system that grows only in its embeddedness within the human world of language and interpersonal relationships. Therefore, neuroscience joins with phenomenology's insistence that to understand a person, even at the level of neurological functioning, typically requires an exploration of the person's world of experience (Adams 2020).

Neuroscience may be on the verge of giving the DSM an alternative perceptual view of diagnosis with such instruments as PET scans, MRIs, and CTs and mindfulness research. It looks promising regarding phenomenology and neuroscience research that studies the experience of neuron movement through electrical circuitry in the brain and combining it with phenomenological experiences in real life. Phenomenology offers a methodically developed theory of human subjectivity that is indispensable to any attempt to understand, explore, and treat psychiatric disorders (Taylor 1971). Psychiatry needs to regain a feeling of "humanity," that is based on observation (outer-viewing), introspection (inner-viewing), and dialogue (interviewing) (Fuchs 2019). This vision is not anti-scientific, but together with the progresses of neuroscience allows an approach based on the whole person (Parnas 2002). A uniquely innovative model for what is happening neurologically in the brain by matching what is happening phenomenologically in a client's experience may become the whole person model of mental health diagnosis. This would be a different option than trying to match neuroscience with a statistical-oriented, a label-oriented, DSM. The reciprocal combination of both experiences appears a reasonable alternative as much as matching neuroscience to a professional collection of observed behaviors and symptoms.

In spite of the lack of hard science, experiential therapists still can have clients describe their traumatic experiences and help them become aware of what is happening in their brains. No matter how primitive and unscientific these descriptions may appear during therapy, they still present a level of effectiveness for motivated clients. Neuroscience gives experiential thinkers the opportunity for a more accurate description of client experiences. This asks the question, whether psychological diagnosis should rely only on a statistical probability of symptoms? Or, should neuroscience research combined with personal experience develop a more experiential/neurological diagnosis? A diagnosis not only grounded in probability but in the possibility of what clients are uniquely "going through" both neurologically and experientially. A uniquely more personal diagnosis than statistical probability based on what patients "have inside of them" identified by a more standardized label.

NEUROSCIENCE AND PHENOMENOLOGICAL THINKING

Neuroscience is more about an experience than a label. It seems advantageous to diagnose from the "neurological inner experience" of the client and combine this with the client's "phenomenological outer experience." Such a method would be uniquely closer to each client's real-life experience than an abstract label that stands as a probable guess based on an accumulation of other client/patient experiences. It would eliminate the stigma associated with labeling disorders that may impact client identity, possibly for the rest of their lives, while fitting more closely with the practices found in physical medicine.

If you have cancer, the focus is not on recognizing it by going to a book based on statistical probability of cancer symptoms to render a diagnosis. In physical medicine, a doctor would directly deal with the experiences your body is going through. The doctor might prescribe a blood test, maybe order an MRI, or possibly perform a biopsy to see if your body is showing signs of cancerous activity. From this direct information, the medical doctor forms a diagnosis around these actual, experiential results. All of these procedures are direct actions that become a patient's unique profile or chart, and not a standardized form of diagnosis emanating from a book based on cancer, even when learning about cancer is important. At some point, one may learn about how cancer looks and works, but for the patient's unique experience with cancer, the medical doctor wants to visualize how cancer is dynamically affecting this patient's body—some patients have a higher tolerance for cancer, and some do not, and so on.

Mental health professionals would like to perform the same procedures with mental disorders. However, as of this writing, neuroscience has not reached the point where professionals can be specific enough, for example, to pinpoint the brain circuitry that causes the experience of depression. To visualize how depression is dynamically affecting the client's neurological and experiential style of depression. Yet, for an experiential therapist both neuroscience and phenomenology hold great importance in understanding a client more holistically.

When clients are telling a story based on eminently personal traumatic events, the therapist can still help them, in more layman's terms, by becoming aware of the trauma within their real-life stories, and combining them with a description of what is happening within the circuitry of the brain (Ladd 2018). It becomes the described neurological effects of trauma that adds credence to the client's traumatic story. It supplies the client with a more holistic and neurological understanding of their experience. It adds meaning and helps in creating trust in the therapeutic process by combining neuroscience with phenomenology. It joins knowledge with wisdom where a client can gain access to the workings of the brain while simultaneously connecting this knowledge to the wisdom found in actual experiences.

So, what would be the value in making the unconscious circuitry in the client's brain more available through mental health therapy? The value may be best expressed not in the brain but in the client's mind. The traditional view of the mind revolves around the belief in mental health that in understanding mental disorders, the mind is directly connected to the brain, and it is this "closed system" between brain and mind that causes mental disorders (Siegel 2016). In psychiatry this view of the mind supports the use of psychotropic drugs as a remedy where drugs are used to change brain chemistry which results in symptoms reduction, ultimately affecting the patient's mind. Or, through a patient's disorganized mind that will eventually have a negative impact regarding the patient's brain, such as expressed in therapy techniques like CBT. This oversimplified but accepted description points out a traditional view of the brain/mind relationship, and helps to justify the current procedures used in the medical model, where symptoms reduction is the ultimate goal, and where psychotropic drugs and cognitive-oriented techniques are commonplace in making the reduction of these symptoms (Perry 2016).

A more progressive, neurological/experiential picture of the mind emerges out of a more holistic view. In this perspective, energy and information flows from our real-life experiences, along with our whole body and brain absorbing this energy and information, where the combination of human experiences and neurological experiences self-organize and emerge in what we call the mind (Siegel 2010). In this "open system of the mind" life experiences have equal importance as the whole body and brain in forming the workings of the mind. A compelling development in accepting this vision of the mind happened through the discovery of neuroplasticity, and how neural pathways can be altered through human experience, especially human relationships (Kays et al. 2012). This view of the mind has given credibility to the power of dialogue in helping clients grow and change, both neurologically and experientially. For the experiential therapist, any description of how brain circuitry works regarding the client's traumatic experiences adds meaning to their story and the therapy process. The traumatic story becomes not only a story of trauma but an internal part of how the brain functions when under trauma. (This process can be observed in the practice of trauma-informed care therapy.) Such a combination helps clients form an expertise in their own recovery. For the experiential thinker in mental health, the belief behind such a practice is not centered on medical model symptoms reduction but more on humanistic growth and change. Anytime therapists can help educate clients neurologically regarding their experiences, points more toward client empowerment and client resilience—an intrinsically valuable process in creating new possibilities for impacting client identity, beyond reducing client symptoms.

CASE STUDY

The case study reflects more of a trauma model that closely aligns with experiential thinking, especially when considering human experience.

Didi was referred to the Trauma Center by an insightful law enforcement officer who was investigating a violent case of rape where she was the victim. The therapist, Tish, was an experiential thinker based on trauma-informed care who did not follow medical model procedures of gathering fact-finding information, making a diagnosis, and coming up with a treatment plan. Except for general statements concerning what happened and how Didi was dealing with it, her major focus was on Didi's safety both physically and emotionally. On the other hand, Didi wanted to gloss over her traumatic history of violence, drugs, and physical and emotional abuse in general terms, basically to inform Tish that she was a tough person and could handle emotionally and psychologically what had happened to her. Her vague list of traumas was her defense against any empathic treatment that Tish may offer her, and she remained silent about sharing her history.

Instead of diving into the rape and former traumatic experiences, Tish asked Didi whether she would like a cup of coffee, and maybe some pastries that she had available. With a certain startled look Didi said, "Why thank you. Yes, please." Tish poured her a cup of coffee and proceeded with small talk which did reveal Didi's love of fashion, and how she liked to read fashion magazines and dream, if she had the money, buying expensive cloths and mixing with others who appreciated fashion.

The next time that Didi saw Tish for therapy, a cup of coffee was awaiting her, along with some interesting pastries. The conversation then turned again to fashion and fashion magazines where Tish asked if she had seen the latest issue of a popular magazine that covered contemporary fashion. As the sessions progressed, Tish would inform Didi that she wanted her to feel comfortable, and that for now her main goal was to help her calm down after such a severe trauma had taken place. Instead of Didi spouting her original mantra about being tough, and that she could handle her trauma, she instead thanked Tish for her honesty and her bluntness in what her intentions were all about. Over time, a certain bond developed between them. This especially was important after the rapist was caught, and depositions from police and lawyers suddenly were asked of her. For the first time, Didi shared with Tish her reluctance in talking about the incident, again for fear that it would bring up traumatic memories.

Finally, Didi said, "I rather tell you first about the incident before I have to bare my soul to outsiders, and to visit again memories of this terrible person who raped me." Tish told Didi that she would speak with the judge and law enforcement about preparing her for these events, so that she was not re-traumatized by the experience. A time line was set for her depositions, and Didi and Tish formed a plan to face the trauma of the event. The plan was to describe the event slowly and only when Didi was ready to share it. Tish thought of an idea to help normalize the experience by having Didi record her story when ready, and playing back the recording to herself, again when ready. At a certain point, she could share it with Tish again when ready, or she could choose to not to share it with her. Tish continuously emphasized that Didi's personal safety was her major concern.

Within the time line designated by the courts, Didi did follow through on the plan; however, she did not at that time want to share her story with Tish. A few weeks passed until the depositions were going to be taken, and Tish prepared Didi by telling her such statements that "you do not have to tell in graphic details if you do not want to." She helped with her breathing, so she would not overreact to the questions asked, and made clear that she would be available after the ordeal of sharing her story was finally over. Didi's appearance before the deposition and eventually her appearance in court left her exhausted but somewhat normalized with Tish's help.

After the appearances with depositions and court appearances a shift seemed to take place in Didi. She described feeling like a raw nerve that wanted to burst through her body and escape her former life, but she was not sure that sharing it was worth the trouble. Tish decided to help Didi with the importance of sharing, again when ready, by giving her insight into what happens neurologically under trauma. She asked Didi's permission if that would be helpful and Didi immediately agreed. Whether Didi's agreement was to distract away from former emotions involved in trauma or was a valid attempt to understand what neurological effects trauma had on her body and brain was unclear. Yet in either case, Tish intuitively felt it was a healthy idea.

In the next session, Tish showed her a diagram of the human brain, pointing out the different regions, but mostly focused on the limbic region where emotions are the main function. She pointed out the amygdala (crisis center), hippocampus (memory center), and how trauma disrupts the memory center by not being able to effectively file away traumatic memories so, to a certain degree, they stay open and can be affected by the crisis center when similar traumas are experienced in one's life (Duckworth 2015). She also talked about the dissociation that happens when trauma is continuously present, and how one dissociates as protection from traumatic personal feelings. She gave Didi some of the physical consequences of trauma by describing the hypothalamus-pituitary-adrenal axis or HPA that leads to insomnia, autoimmune disorders, and digestive disorders (Banitt 2018).

Didi informed Tish that the information was like describing her life experiences down to the most vital detail. It gave her insight that pulled together many of the traumatic experiences that she went through during the course of her life. It gave her a reason to begin sharing all those traumas that preceded the rape incident. Tish and Didi began working through former traumas by having a meaningful dialogue, then using EMDR techniques to help normalize them—always appreciating the positive regard that made Didi feel safe, and by recognizing the bond between them.

DISCUSSION

Medical model decision-making is more through calculations in therapy, whereas experiential thinkers tend to be intuitive in their decisions during therapy. This is exemplified in the case study, where Tish intuitively realized that Didi was not ready for any discussion of the traumatic rape incident. Instead, she intuitively asked her whether she would like coffee. Based on Tish's main belief that safety is the most pressing concern, she intuitively and intentionally asked Didi whether coffee would make her feel safe and comfortable without actually explaining her intentions. This was not a calculation, but an intuition that neurologically has a more complicated neural structure than any logical, calculated decision. First, intuitive decisions are more quickly made, and may be responsible for our survival over the past 50,000 years because they happen without thinking. It is the ventromedial prefrontal cortex that can elicit the emotional responses that people deem as gut feelings or hunches (Bechara, Damasion, Damasion and Gregory 1999). Combine this with the locus ceruleus, a minute nucleus located in the pons in the middle brain, and this combination is said to generate one's gut feelings. The reason is that the pons area supplies noradrenaline to the forebrain, which influences emotion, motivation, memory, learning, and decision-making, and because of this, it also plays a role in the experience of intuition (Demasio 2005). Most neuroscientists view intuition as condensed reasoning or swift cognition—a person's ability to exploit the brain's shortcuts (Fiora 2017). An experiential thinker believes in staying as much in the present moment as possible with the intention of making emotional contact with a client.

Phenomenologist call this a disciplined naivete—the ability to clear your mind of judgments, and simply focus on what is in front of you (Merleau-Ponty 2002). Practitioners of mindfulness espouse a similar practice. I personally call this, "We let the outside world rewire our brains without our input." In the field of trauma therapy, such a belief seems mandatory especially when a trauma victim is in crisis. Nowhere in the techniques for dealing with trauma is having a cup of coffee and a pastry a formal therapy technique. However, it is that exact moment of intuitive decision-making where Tish used the coffee/pastry form of therapy to offer Didi an expression of safety—a nuanced gesture with enormous neurological and experiential impact, no matter how mundane it may appear. For the experiential therapist, intuitive decisions align more closely with an open, free-flowing dialogue between client and therapist.

Neurologically, there are other reasons why experiential therapists may hold more value in this form of therapy, especially in trauma therapy. In experiential therapy, attunement or emotionally connecting is an essential component both neurologically and experientially. As talk therapists, when interacting with clients, mirror neurons are activated in our brains, by reading a client's body language, gestures, posture, and tone of voice. These experiences create emotional meaning in the therapist and client. Neurologically, it is the mirror neurons that are responsible for this activity. Neuroscientists have stated that they are the only brain cells we know of that seem specialized in coding the actions of other people, and also our own actions (Iacobini 2009). They become the essential brain cells for any social interactions.

How important was it for Tish to make a firm emotional connection or attunement with Didi? Attunement along with making moment-to-moment intuitive decisions may be the therapy difference in effectively helping victims of trauma, or any other client-oriented mental problem. Didi being emotionally dissociated or numb to her feelings, and eventually forming an emotional attachment with Tish, can be the foundation for future growth and change. The ability to have empathic reactions to other people's pain is a fundamental premise for all talk therapy. A classic medical model recognizes empathy in its training, but in actual practice, it tends to frown on empathy when it takes the client/therapist in different directions then agreed upon in the treatment plan. In some cases, it rather relies on the professional indifference associated with the dissemination of psychotropic drugs, than take the time to connect emotionally with patients.

The combination of empathy, intuition, and attuned connections can lead the client and therapist into making insightful discoveries. This happens when signals in the right superior-temporal gyrus transmits through the right anterior superior-temporal lobe a gamma response. High-frequency oscillation in the right superior-temporal gyrus is the neural calling card for insight. For those non-neuroscientists, this translates into portions of the brain coming together. Not through calculated thought, but through intuitive, empathic, and attuned connections creating that "aha moment" in therapy. Didi experienced insight, when after being subjected to law enforcement and the courts, she had insight into the gravity of her history of traumatic experiences. At that moment she wanted Tish to help her work through these traumas. There is limited rational thought going into these moments. For example, Albert Einstein did not invent $E = mc^2$ from hours of calculation. He discovered it by attending to this meaningful project for years until one day it popped out in an "aha moment." His prior knowledge and intuitive ability made it eventually reveal itself, much in the same fashion as Didi's trauma popped out and wanted to be revealed.

Again, in a comparison between experiential thinking and medical model thinking, the issue of trust versus control returns as an important theme.

The experiential thinking of Tish trusted the wisdom found in attunement, intuition, empathy, and insight. The calculations found in a medical model's reliance on seeking a logical outcome based on a treatment plan and by controlling the data seems a cumbersome way of revealing actual mental health problems to many professionals who rely on their intuition to give direction in therapy.

When we usually think about neuroscience and its connection to mental health, psychotropic drug research seems the common connection between the two. This chapter demonstrates a connection still exists, but it is not necessarily in neurological research with psychotropic drugs. Neuroscience is more focused on neurological circuitry in the brain than developing new drugs for mental health. The current focus in neuroscience seems more amenable to phenomenological (experiential) research, where the inner workings of the brain compliment the outer workings of client's experience. Time will tell whether research combines these dynamic fields of thought.

These new developments hopefully will increase the awareness for empirically oriented therapists who perceive some experiential therapists as the "poets in psychology."

Demonstrating the neurological benefits of experience-oriented skills such as intuition, empathy, attunement, and insight can offer the mental health profession a viable alternative to a strict medical model. Also, even though experiential therapy may not reflect the guidelines followed in empiricism, it may hold weight in the field of neuroscience. A future is opened for the creation of a new neurological/experiential method of diagnosis.

There is no question whether reliance on statistical probability and the standardization of mental disorders through the DSM has benefited the field of mental health. It remains the foundation of the profession's business portion of the practice, where insurance companies and drug companies have concerted interest in keeping mental disorders in linear categories, where one disorder is clearly separate from another—not to mention the cluster of symptoms identification that helps designate a psychological label. In response, the more holistic, experiential therapists appear better-equipped if and when the time arrives that neuroscience is sophisticated enough to isolate mental disorders through brain circuitry. The future looks promising for those who believe that neuroscience and human experience should holistically work together.

NOTE

1. This gives an indication of where neuroscience is headed regarding mental health diagnosis. I have stated since 2012 that phenomenological experiences were a

better vehicle for collaboration regarding mental disorders than statistical probability. "Where is Mental Health Diagnosis Heading, And Where Does the DSM Fall Short?" (Ladd 2012).

It proves to me that the "business" of mental health holds precedence over the therapeutic process. George Engel. 1997. "From Biomedical to Biopsychosocial: Being Scientific in the Human Condition," *Psychodynamic Psychiatry* 40 (3): 377–96 and (Peter Ladd. 2012. "Where Is Mental Health Diagnosis Heading, and Where Does the DSM Fall Short?" *Institute of Mental Health* 29 (June).

Chapter 14

The Experiential Therapist

It would be safe to say that for the therapy discussed in this book, client experience matters. The previous chapters point out the importance of personal experience in mental health therapy, and therapists may need a specific attitude in therapy to capture these experiences. There are very few therapy experts or anyone else, who understand the depth of the experiences of clients, even though clients are most affected by their input. The attitude of the experiential therapist in this book is more holistic than empirical. Seeing client's problems from a holistic perspective opens up possibilities from many different angles for personal healing. An experiential therapist may start by talking about feelings, or discussing neuroscience, or having a dialogue over how one thinks about pain and suffering or focus on techniques that may change that thinking. In experiential therapy, procedures for what happens, unfold in real time, and procedures are always different, depending on the experiences of each client. This is the major contrast between medical model mental health therapists and experiential therapists. The medical model therapist follows procedures that, for the most part, are standardized while the experiential therapist creates a series of personalized experiences fashioned around the dialogue between client and therapist.

What becomes more standardized in experience is the creative approach taken in understanding what clients are going through regarding their pain and suffering. Mental health therapy from an experiential approach is *not* primarily focused on standardized procedures, but on more *real-time beliefs* regarding what is the most effective method for helping clients. I have tried to capture some of these beliefs and wanted to present them in a more comparison fashion for those readers, who desire a synthesized collection of the basic approaches taken with an experiential therapist. Primarily, the idea of therapy is not in the hands of an expert, but in the dialogue between client and therapist. For those of you who want to continue the journey into experiential therapy, I reference the book that precedes the present book called *The Talk Therapy Revolution: Neuroscience, Phenomenology and Mental Health.*

COLLABORATION

One of the reasons for using a collaboration format in experiential therapy is to introduce another perspective of how clients see their experiences. This is a more phenomenological approach to mental health therapy where the therapist is not trying to match client experience with the DSM of Mental Disorders but is attempting to find common ground between the therapist's perspective on the mental problem with the client's perspective. These two perspectives, one for the client's awareness of the experience and the therapist's point of view, give a more well-rounded and holistic understanding—one that has a more comprehensive perspective not an empirical analysis. Also, collaboration helps to break down walls between therapist and client through forming a therapeutic alliance, so what is shared is a dialogue that most accurately tries to identify the problem.

Collaboration gives value to the learned experience in therapy. It makes the pain and suffering a part of the client's story, giving negative experiences within the client's story purpose and meaning. When therapists collaborate with clients, both learn from each other their mistakes, successes, and commitments. Collaboration tends to raise the mood of clients, so important before a therapeutic alliance can be formed. They feel that someone is on their side and has their back. From such a stance can arise a climate of trust that is different than medical model emphasis on control and is opposed to an expert that is going to cure them.

An atmosphere where collaboration is front and center in therapy is important for the client/therapist experience, and it will go a long way toward preventing them from making assumptions about the suffering on their own. Connection matters in therapy. I believe that clients want to work with people they trust, who understand and respect different points of view, and who work well together. Collaboration lays the foundation for a more open, connected, and engaged therapy. Simply put, working collaboratively makes healing possible. Collaboration is a part of a professional culture that values experience, and this has a ripple effect when being a successful collaborator where clients then tend to collaborate with others outside the therapy experience.

WISDOM

Knowledge is retained. Wisdom is obtained through experience. In the dynamics of experiential therapy, the therapist relies on wisdom more than knowledge. In traditional medical model mental health therapy, one takes the knowledge learned and applies it through specific procedures. It is the procedures themselves that are supposed to direct the patient toward symptom reduction and symptom maintenance. In experiential therapy, wisdom is not set in standardized procedures, but is found in either client or the therapist's former experiences, or in the practice of former knowledge obtained during one's education. Therefore, you can be knowledgeable as a therapist, but there is no guarantee you are effective. It is through experience of making mistakes and having successes that wisdom forms in the minds of effective experiential therapists.

One other phenomenon that applies to wisdom is when therapists make more intuitive decisions than calculated decisions. Through successes, mistakes, and practice, the therapist obtains a different sense of what is happening with the client. Experiential therapists do not attempt a perception of symptoms to justify a diagnosis but observe important nuances that signal purpose and meaning are happening. This usually ensues after a therapist forms a therapeutic alliance, where the connection is made more through intuition than calculation. Where a bond is created where both client and therapist trust, where the dialogue around positive and negative experiences will take them. Wisdom directs the therapy not through standardized procedures but through instinct, intuition, and insight. These phenomena are more closely aligned with the actual experience of the client.

NEUROSCIENCE

Neuroscience has increasingly become a part of experiential thinking in mental health therapy. Phenomenology is about capturing the *outer* experiences that clients are going through, and to help them successfully work through these experiences. Neuroscience from an experiential perspective is capturing the *inner* experience that clients are going through by changing the negative neuropathways that cause the client's negative experiences. It is this combination that gives neuroscience a place in phenomenological thinking. Before neuroscience, phenomenology (the study of experience) was on its own trying to demonstrate the importance of focusing on experience in mental health therapy. Since MRIs, PET scans, and others, one sees the impact that negative experiences have on the brain (Litrell 2015). Therefore, negative neuropathways can lead to negative experiences, and negative experiences can reinforce negative pathways in the brain.

This also is an opportunity for experience to join forces with empiricism, in order to give a more holist view of client problems without empirical, natural scientific procedures monopolizing the therapy process. Experiential therapy tries to be as comprehensive as possible, so including neuroscience as one other perspective of human experience is a more exacting way to pinpoint a client's reality. In many respects, experience needs neuroscience to be a legitimate possibility for all those empirically minded therapists where efficacy reins over effectiveness. Conversely, neuroscience needs experience to check on the effectiveness of neurological changes during actual client experiences. On the other hand, medical model mental health therapy does not rely on experience or neuroscience as methods for developing diagnoses and treatment plans. They are grounded in the results of statistics and professional observation. I believe we will see in the future a more accepted connection between experience and neuroscience in understanding client disorders, only in a more reciprocal relationship, not dominated by natural science, so ubiquitously found in modernist beliefs.

PATTERNS

A comparison between experiential patterns and medical model labels reveals some obvious differences. First, let us look at medical model labels. It is true that labels in mental health therapy makes it easier to communicate with other professionals in the field of mental health, but experiential patterns make it easier to communicate with clients. If clients are looking to find information on a specific mental disorder regarding what is wrong with them, labels will fulfill that need better than patterns. Labels are also a way to describe a problem without getting into detail. Unfortunately, labels can become stereotypical when it comes to personal identity. For example, I am bipolar.

Once you tell someone your label, it has a tendency to categorize and identify you by the label. Experiential patterns describe what you are going through. Instead of identifying yourself, you are in a better position to get outside yourself and compare one's experiences with experiences of others with no pattern being exactly the same. Patterns give personalized road maps that help clients work through these experiences. Also, labels can help clients avoid their experiences by saying such things as, "Don't ask me to do anything I am bi-polar."

The other issue with experiential patterns is they are designed to give the essence or the basic series of events an intentional direction, for example, "In your experience you started out feeling frustrated, and then your frustration led to feeling stuck, so you buried your frustration, until you could not keep it buried, then you began to lash out at everyone and now they think you have a behavioral problem. We need to find a way to unstick you from your frustration." These and any number of other patterns give the client a series of events that they can understand rather, in the above example simply saying, "You have oppositional defiant disorder."

DIALOGUE

Dialogue along with empathy and creating a therapeutic alliance may be three of the most important phenomena in experiential therapy. Unlike debate, dialogue does not involve arguing for a point of view, defending a set of assumptions as in medical model mental health therapy, or critiquing the positions of others. Unlike negotiation or consensus-building, it's not a method of reaching agreement or arriving at decisions. And unlike discussion, it can only emerge when participants trust and respect each other, suspend their judgments, and listen deeply to all points of view. The purpose is not so much to solve a problem or resolve an issue as to explore the most promising avenues for action (London 2018). Under these premises, dialogue explores possibilities wherever the experience being presented takes both client and therapist. It becomes the creative source of healing within the intuitive decisions being made by both parties for eventual growth and change.

I believe that dialogue can get lost when therapists become overly responsible for diagnoses, labels, and treatment plans. These predetermined guidelines leave little room for dialogue to eventually lead us to wisdom and insight. These are two phenomena that do not follow any given plan. They emerge out of the creative dialogue between two people with different perspectives, trying to reach a particular place of clarity. When dialogue is effective both empathy and forming a therapeutic alliance between client and therapist becomes a more natural process. When too many guidelines and procedures enter therapy the chances of an effective dialogue diminishes. They flatten the complexity for the sake of diagnosis, undermining a holistic, humanistic, and a nuanced approach. The procedures followed in medical model therapy tend to be less of an opportunity for dialogue, even though it may not be intentional.

SUFFERING

Pain is inevitable. Suffering is optional. In experiential mental health therapy, there is a distinction between necessary and unnecessary suffering. In a medical model form of mental health therapy, the idea is to get rid of all suffering connected to disorders through symptom reduction. This is based on patients viewing their suffering as a part of a disorder. When you critically think through what is happening in a medical model, it may appear there is confusion between pain and suffering. Pain is inevitable and to reduce pain makes sense in therapy. In experiential therapy suffering becomes optional. A client can choose to suffer at the passing of a loved one out of respect for that person, no matter how painful the experience. Or, a client may choose not to suffer the pain connected to severe anxiety by mindfulness training or psychotropic drugs. In some cases, suffering through an experience can reduce the pain connected to suffering—as in a traumatic incident of abuse. By taking a stand and reclaiming one's dignity may require suffering to alleviate the pain. Suffering and pain are better defined in experiential therapy based on talking through experiences where a client can find purpose and meaning for suffering. This is opposed to a medical model where a patient understands he or she has a painful disorder and needs to rid one's self of the pain. In experiential thinking, pain is inevitable, but suffering becomes a choice based on whether in life experiences it appears necessary or unnecessary. Beyond this is experiential thinking that believes that necessary suffering creates resilience and courage that should not be denied a client's chances for growth and change.

NUANCES

In mental health therapy, nuances describe something that has subtle, complex shades of meaning and understanding. Nuances are very small expressions of meaning that include behaviors, perceptions, understanding, or appearance that provide deep insights into the complex nature of human experience. Therapy is rarely a black or white experience, and, for example, medical model mental health therapy is not based on facts but on probabilities. Being able to think and understand experiences in nuanced ways can be beneficial to the therapeutic process. This may be why experiential therapists focus on nuances more than psychological symptoms. In experiential therapy, the therapist practices and tries to be disciplined in picking out the nuances when a client responds during the dialogue between therapist and client. The belief is that nuances accurately capture how the client is feeling or thinking at that moment, and in that moment such nuances may stand for a more meaningful reality facing the client's problems.

Nuances may help the therapist discover the deeper changes that clients and therapists are looking for when in dialogue with each other. In medical model therapy, these deeper changes may be missed based on a therapist that is focusing mostly on client symptoms, which have become standardized in the DSM. This takes away the importance of those moment-to-moment nuances that may stand for deeper meaning that specifically describes client suffering, but also can help in an awareness of client recovery. A client demonstrated symptoms of anxiety, but during therapy showed subtle nuances of betrayal by a loved one. For the experiential therapist, treating only the anxiety is a superficial solution of a far deeper problem based on betrayal. Following the nuances down to uncovering those moments of betrayal may have meaning for client recovery, and along the way, may defuse the symptoms of anxiety. Just treating only the anxiety may leave the underlying meaning of betrayal untouched.

MOMENTUM

Momentum may be the most accurate method for evaluating success in mental health therapy for the experiential therapist. This is not the case for the medical model therapist, who evaluates success by how much change takes place in reducing the symptoms of a disorder. If symptoms are reduced, then the therapy has been successful. These are the same guidelines for the use of psychotropic drugs. Symptom reduction followed by symptom maintenance measures success by the therapist, and not to mention for the pharmaceutical companies.

For the experiential therapist who is more dedicated to listening to client experiences, momentum is more the measure of success and failure. If a client comes to therapy with extreme negative momentum regarding depression, one of the responsibilities of the experiential therapist is to try and turn that momentum around to something more positive. This usually begins by forming therapeutic alliances with the client. Here is a simple analogy to describe when an experiential therapist is successful in therapy.

If you decide to roll a small snowball down a hill, you will have to roll it yourself until it becomes big enough that it will move on its own momentum. For experiential therapists, one remains dedicated to the client until she or he has gained enough momentum that the therapeutic services are no longer needed. The client has gained enough momentum to face their problems on their own. Another way of saying this is when clients feel empowered enough and have gained enough momentum, they are ready to resume an unencumbered creative lifestyle. It becomes the responsibility of the therapist to help create momentum for the client. It becomes the responsibility of the client to keep the momentum going. This may be why medical model success with clients is based on symptom reduction where it may or may not provide enough momentum for patients to keep being successful without the help of the medical model therapist.

DWELLING

Dwelling in experiential therapy is the process whereby a client concentrates on some feature of their experiential mental problem at the exclusion of other's portions of the problem. For example, a client realizes in therapy that he or she needs to move on from the habitual pattern of worrying. They do this not by ruminating on the problem, but by concentrating on specific future possibilities not through calculated thinking but more from an intuitive dwelling or meditation on those future possibilities. In essence, dwelling is a form of meditation where there is no goal or problem to be resolved, but an awareness of trusting the process that some insight or "aha moment" will emerge.

Dwelling sometimes becomes confused with ruminating or worrying when a client tries to solve their problems by thinking over and over again with no success in solving anything except a possible increase in anxiety. In order to dwell in experiential therapy, it is important that both client and therapist retreat from the empirical mind's need to calculate an answer. In experience, trying to control how to face suffering and pain by setting goals and calculating guidelines is unnecessary. Problem-solving answers are replaced with dialogue that relies on wisdom, nuances, and momentum to develop an attitude where answers emerge on their own. Dwelling as a theme of experience has become more popular in recent years based on its association with mindfulness, and its close association with meditation. Both require non-calculated thinking, and both require the ability to dwell on one theme, and when distracted to return back to that theme.

FLEXIBILITY

Flexibility in mental health therapy is a primary factor in resilience, and is reflective of an individual's emotional adjustment and maturity. Flexibility also ensures in therapy that some form of hope will eventually emerge if the client practices resilience. One of the problems facing the medical model therapist is how to incorporate flexibility into a fairly rigid scientific method. Not having the flexibility to fit a new direction for the patient in therapy changes any new directional technique in therapy that must fit the scientific method. Experientially based therapy has the advantage of changing directions in therapy at any point in the dialogue between client and therapist, when the dialogue calls for a change, thus developing empowerment within the client. The burden of sticking by a preconceived diagnosis or treatment plan is eliminated through the free-flowing nature of following the client's experiences wherever they may lead the therapy process.

It may be that such flexibility in the experiential style of therapy at times can be a challenge for the novice therapists, but for the experienced therapists, it hopefully gives the opportunity for more consistent accuracy when working with clients. It also points out for experienced therapists when it might be time to refer a case to another professional, when the flexibility in the therapist's methods is not making progress or creating results. One of the problems with some clients who come to therapy is that they may have a specific problem with, for example, depression, but their secondary problem may be the inability to be flexible when searching for methods of recovery. If you can get over a mental problem in a day, week, or month, one still has a certain amount of flexibility to recover. If it is taking a year, five years or more, then part of your problem may be your inability to be flexible.

OWNERSHIP

It is one thing to learn new skills in mental health and within a month or two have those skills abandoned because in the everyday practice of therapy they lose their meaning. They have yet to become a part of one's everyday practice. In a sense, the client has rented them and has yet to own them where practicing a distinct skill has yet to become a part one's specific style of recovery. Ownership of skills may require a therapist to go to higher levels of learning beyond memory, comprehension, and application. To own a mental health skill, it may require the client to analyze, synthesize, and self-evaluate whether this skill will become a part of one's overall style of recovery. Without such a learned response learning skills and techniques remain only information to be aware of but not necessarily practiced day in and day out. The level of information to choose from in the mental health profession is staggering. Unless these skills have personal ownership by the client, they may simply fall into the memory banks of aware information.

LAST THOUGHTS

I have tried to capture some of the phenomena that make up the identity of an experiential therapist. In previous books, I have discussed other experiential themes that help define one's role in experiential thinking. In this book, I believe enough has been covered to understand the difference between these two models. This is not to say that all mental health therapists should consider finding their identity in experience. There are many variables to consider including your attitude toward practicing an expertise or collaborating with clients, what you value more, knowledge or wisdom, your approach to a reciprocal form of neuroscience, your interest in patterns over labels, your ability to create a dialogue rather than give directions, your sense of flexibility or control, your ability to attend rather than calculate, and your comfort level with momentum over procedures. Also included in making a decision to be more experiential is the nature of your work environment, the attitudes of your colleagues, weighing having a job, as opposed to having an ideological perspective, the resilience needed to go against the predominate culture of the medical model, and how much your experiences have influenced your identity. Being an experiential therapist is an alternative way of thinking about the profession of mental health therapy. It continues to offer some creative possibilities, while at the same time offering some challenging roadblocks. Yet, in the twenty-first century, I believe, we have a chance to move away from an outlook in the mental health profession, based only on the scientific method of standardization, and include a more experiential perspective based on a diversity of options given to each client in therapy. I as write this the world of mental health is changing. It may be perceptions of mental illness will begin to broaden where client/patients are not only viewed as sick but also as injured from life experiences. In my long-standing practice, only some of these issues have been answered regarding my personal perspective about this profession such as "how difficult is it to change the culture of mental health?" or "will the momentum of the information age make that decision for us?" So, my intent in writing in this book, hopefully will give you some answers to what approach is valid for you. More importantly, I hope this writing has clarified some of the questions involved in practicing mental health therapy from an experiential perspective.

Glossary

ACT

Developed within a coherent theoretical and philosophical framework, Acceptance and Commitment Therapy (ACT) is a unique empirically based psychological intervention that uses acceptance and mindfulness strategies, together with commitment and behavior change strategies, to increase psychological flexibility.

Aha Movments

The eureka effect (also known as the Aha! moment or eureka moment) refers to the common human experience of suddenly understanding a previously incomprehensible problem or concept. Some research describes the Aha! . . . First, the Aha!

Catastrophizing

Catastrophizing is an irrational thought a lot of us have in believing that something is far worse than it actually is. Catastrophizing can generally take two different forms: making a catastrophe out of a current situation and imagining making a catastrophe out of a future situation.

Cognitive Behavioral Therapy

Cognitive behavioral therapy (CBT) is a short-term, goal-oriented psychotherapy treatment that takes a hands-on, practical approach to problem-solving. Its goal is to change patterns of thinking or behavior that are behind people's difficulties, and so change the way they feel.

Disciplined Naivete

Phenomenology for acts as well as content; it is a tolerant discipline. European phrasing is more extreme: French psychologist Merleau-Ponty says, "The whole effort is to recover naive contact with the world."

DSM 5

The *Diagnostic and Statistical Manual of Mental Disorders, Fifth Edition* (DSM-5) is the 2013 update to the *Diagnostic and Statistical Manual of Mental Disorders*, the taxonomic and diagnostic tool published by the American Psychiatric Association (APA). In the United States, the DSM serves as the principal authority for psychiatric diagnoses. Treatment recommendations, as well as payment by health care providers, are often determined by DSM classifications, so the appearance of a new version has significant practical importance.

EMDR

EMDR (Eye Movement Desensitization and Reprocessing) is a psychotherapy that enables people to heal from the symptoms and emotional distress that are the result of disturbing life experiences. Repeated studies show that by using EMDR therapy people can experience the benefits of psychotherapy that once took years to make a difference. It is widely assumed that severe emotional pain requires a long time to heal. EMDR therapy shows that the mind can in fact heal from psychological trauma much as the body recovers from physical trauma. When you cut your hand, your body works to close the wound. If a foreign object or repeated injury irritates the wound, it festers and causes pain. Once the block is removed, healing resumes. EMDR therapy demonstrates that a similar sequence of events occurs with mental processes. The brain's information processing system naturally moves toward mental health. If the system is blocked or imbalanced by the impact of a disturbing event, the emotional wound festers and can cause intense suffering. Once the block is removed, healing resumes. Using the detailed protocols and procedures learned in EMDR therapy training sessions, clinicians help clients activate their natural healing processes.

Emotional Intelligence

Emotional intelligence (EI), emotional leadership (EL), emotional quotient (EQ) and emotional intelligence quotient (EIQ) is the capability of individuals to recognize their own emotions and those of others, discern between different feelings and label them appropriately, use emotional information to guide thinking and behavior, and manage and/or adjust emotions to adapt to environments or achieve one's goal.

Hippocampus

Hippocampus, region of the brain that is associated primarily with memory. The name *hippocampus* is derived from the Greek *hippokampus* (*hippos*, meaning "horse," and *kampos*, meaning "sea monster"), since the structure's shape resembles that of a seahorse. The hippocampus, which is located in the inner (medial) region of the temporal lobe, forms part of the limbic system, which is particularly important in regulating emotional responses. The hippocampus is thought to be principally involved in storing long-term memories and in making those memories resistant to forgetting, though this is a matter of debate. It is also thought to play an important role in spatial processing and navigation.

International Classification of Disease (ICD-11)

The World Health Organization (WHO) is today releasing its new International Classification of Diseases (ICD-11). The ICD is the foundation for identifying health trends and statistics worldwide, and contains around 55,000 unique codes for injuries, diseases, and causes of death.

Lexapro

Lexapro (escitalopram) is a type of antidepressant called a selective serotonin reuptake inhibitor (SSRI) used to treat anxiety in adults and major depressive disorder in adults and adolescents who are at least twelve years old.

Limbic System

The limbic system is a complex set of structures that lies on both sides of the thalamus, just under the cerebrum. It includes the hypothalamus, the hippocampus, the amygdala, and several other nearby areas.

Locus Coeruleus

The primary function of the locus coeruleus is to regulate the amount of noradrenaline in the forebrain. Thus, at a behavioral or systems level, the function of the locus coeruleus critically depends upon the dynamic interaction between the released noradrenaline and neuronal activity in its multiple target areas.

Natural Scientific Methodology

Natural science is a branch of science concerned with the description, prediction, and understanding of natural phenomena, based on empirical evidence from observation and experimentation. Mechanisms such as peer review and repeatability of findings are used to try to ensure the validity of scientific advances.

Neural Networks

A neural network is an artificial network or mathematical model for information processing based on how neurons and synapses work in the human brain. Using the human brain as a model, a neural network connects simple nodes (or "neurons," or "units") to form a network of nodes—thus the term "neural network."

Neural Pathways

A neural pathway is the connection formed by axons that project from neurons to make synapses onto neurons in another location, to enable a signal to be sent from one region of the nervous system to another. Neurons are connected by a single axon, or by a bundle of axons known as a nerve tract.

Neuroplasticity

Neuroplasticity, also known as brain plasticity, neuro-elasticity, or neural plasticity, is the ability of the brain to change continuously throughout an individual's life, for example, brain activity associated with a given function can be transferred to a different location, the proportion of grey matter can change, and synapses may strengthen or weaken over time. The aim of neuroplasticity is to optimize the neural networks during phylogenesis, ontogeny, and physiological learning, as well as after a brain injury. Research in the latter half of the twentieth century showed that many aspects of the brain can be altered (or are "plastic") even through adulthood. However, the developing brain exhibits a higher degree of plasticity than the adult brain.

PET Scans

A positron emission tomography *(PET) scan* is an imaging test that helps reveal how your tissues and organs are functioning. A *PET scan* uses a radioactive drug (tracer) to show this activity.

Prefrontal Cortex

Prefrontal cortex (PFC) is the cerebral cortex covering the front part of the frontal lobe. This brain region has been implicated in planning complex cognitive behavior, personality expression, decision-making, and moderating social behavior.

Prozac

Prozac is an antidepressant. It is mainly used to treat major depression, obsessive-compulsive disorder, and panic disorder. Also known by its generic name, fluoxetine, Prozac is a selective serotonin reuptake inhibitor (SSRI)

Psychotropic Drugs

Psychotropic medication: any medication capable of affecting the mind, emotions, and behavior. Some medications such as lithium, which may be used to treat depression, are psychotropic. Also called a psychodynamic medication.

PTSD

Post-traumatic stress disorder (PTSD) is a mental health condition that is triggered by a terrifying event—either experiencing it or witnessing it. Symptoms may include flashbacks, nightmares, and severe anxiety, as well as uncontrollable thoughts about the event. Most people who go through traumatic events may have temporary difficulty adjusting and coping, but with time and good self-care, they usually get better. If the symptoms get worse, last for months or even years, and interfere with your day-to-day functioning, you may have PTSD.

Schizophreniform Disorder

Schizophreniform disorder is a mental disorder diagnosed when symptoms of schizophrenia are present for a significant portion of the time at least a month, but signs of disturbance are present not for the full six months required for the diagnosis of schizophrenia.

SSRIs

SSRI stands for selective serotonin reuptake inhibitor. SSRI antidepressants are a type of antidepressants that work by increasing levels of serotonin within the brain. Serotonin is a neurotransmitter that is often referred to as the "feel good hormone." It carries messages between brain cells and contributes to well-being, good mood, appetite, as well as helping to regulate the body's sleep-wake cycle and internal clock.

Therapeutic Alliance

The "therapeutic alliance," also called the "therapeutic relationship," is how you and a therapist connect, behave, and engage with each other. Nowadays, the therapeutic alliance is seen by most forms of counseling and psychotherapy as one of the main tools for achieving positive change in the lives of clients.

Bibliography

Abbott, Brianna. 2019. "Deeper Learning." *Natural Medicine* 25 (January): 9–11.

Allsopp, Kate, John Read, Rhiannon Cocoran and Peter Kinbderman. 2019. "Heterogeneity on Psychiatric Diagnostic Classification." *Psychiatry Research* 279, no. 15: 22.

American Psychiatric Association. 2013. *Diagnostic and Statistical Manual 5.* Washington, DC: American Psychological Association.

Banitt, Susan. 2019. *Wisdom Attachment and Love in Trauma Therapy.* New York, NY: Routledge.

Baroud, Ramsey. 2016. "Marketing of Madness: The Truth." *Foreign Policy Journal* 8 (September): 23–27.

Barron, Carrie, 2012. "Sixteen Strategies for Combating Rumination." *Psychology Today,* July 14, 2012.

Barsky, A. 2017. "DSM-5 and the Ethics of Diagnosis." *The New Social Worker Magazine,* April 30, 2017.

Baumeister, David. 2016. "Effects of Psychotropic Drugs on Inflammation: Consequence or Mediator of Therapeutic Effects in Psychiatric Treatment?" *Psychopharmacology* 233, no. 9 (May): 1547–89. doi:10.1007/s00213-015-4044-5

Bechara, Antione, Damasio Hanna, Damasio Antonio, and Lee Gregory. 1990. "Different Contributions of the Human Amygdala and the Ventromedial Prefrontal Cortex to Decision Making." *Social Cognitive and Affective Neuroscience* 7, no. 3 (June): 253–62.

Beidas, Rednad and Phillip Kendall. 2010. "Training Therapists in Evidence-Based Practice: A Critical Review of Studies from a Systems-Contextual Perspective." *Clinical Psychology: Science and Practice* 17: 1–30. doi:10.1111/j.1468-2850.2009. 01187 .x

Bell, Vaughn. 2013. "Changing Brains: Why Neuroscience Is Ending the Prozac Era." *The Guardian*, September 12, 2013.

Benning, Tony. 2015. "Limitations of Bio/psycho/social Model in Psychiatry." *Journal List Advanced Medical Practice* 6: 347–52.

Bien, Thomas. 2006. *Mindful Therapy*. Somerville, MA: Wisdom Publications.
Brown, Hannah. 2012. "How to Stabilize and Acutely Psychotic Patient." *Current Psychiatry* 11, no. 12 (April): 10–16.
Buber, Martin. 2014. *Between Man and Man.* Eastford, CT: Martino Fine Books.
———. 1965. *The Way of Man* (new edition 2002), London: Routledge.
Buckley, Frank. 1971. "Feeling At-Homeness." In Amedeo Giorgi (ed.), *Duquesne Studies in Phenomenological Psychology Vol. 1* (p. 174). Pittsburgh, PA: Duquesne University Press.
Cherry, Kendra. 2019. "What Is Learned Helplessness and Why Does It Happen?" *Very Well Mind,* July 25, 2019.
Chorpita, Bruce, Kimberly Becker and Eric Daleiden. 2007. "Understanding the Common Elements of Evidence-Based Practice: Misconceptions and Clinical Examples." *Journal of the American Academy of Child and Adolescent Psychiatry* 46 (Spring): 647–52. doi:10.1097/chi.0b013e318033ff71
Chung, Man, Bill Fulford and George Graham. 2006. *Re-conceiving Schizophrenia.* Oxford: Oxford University Press.
Cirino, Erica. 2019. "10 Tips to Help You Stop Ruminating." *Healthline,* April: 18.
Coleman, Mark. 2019. *From Suffering to Peace: The True Promise of Mindfulness.* Novato, CA: New World Library.
Collard, D. 2018. "Rigidity versus Flexibility: The Key to Mental Health." *Psychology Central*, October.
Cripps, Charlotte. 2017. "Eurythmics, Nelson Mandela and Global Feminism." *The Circle* 9 (November 9, 2017).
Danchev, Alex. 2013. *The Letters of Paul Cezanne*. Milton Park: Routledge.
Daniels, Jeffery and Lisa Larsen. 2007. "The Impact of Performance Feedback on Counseling Self-efficacy and Counselor Anxiety." *Counselor Education and Supervision* 41 (Fall): 120–30. doi:10.1002/j.1556-6978. 2001. tb01276.x
Deacon, Brett. 2013. "The Biomedical Model of Mental Disorder: A Critical Analysis of Its Validity, Utility, and Effects on Psychotherapy Research." *Psychology Review* 33: 846–61.
deBeer, Wayne. 2017. "Original Opinion: The Use of Bloom's Taxonomy to Teach and Assess the Skill of the Psychiatric Formulation during Vocational Training." *The Royal Australian and New Zealand College of Psychiatrists*, August 31.
Dehaene, Stanislas. 2019. "Touching and Pushing the Limits of the Human Brain." *Edge*, January: 10.
Deurzen, Emmy. 2015. "Phenomenological Therapy." In Edward S. Neukrug (ed.), *Encyclopedia for Counseling and Psychotherapy* (p. 24). Thousand Oaks, CA: Sage Publications.
Dodd, Celia. 2015. "Open Dialogue: The Radical New Treatment Having Life-Changing Effects On People's Mental Health." *Independent Journal* 16: 57.
Duckworth, Ken. 2015. "Science Meets the Human Experience: Integrating the Medical Model and Recovery Model." *National Alliance on Mental Illness*, April 10: 35–45.
Duncan, Barry and Robert Reese. 2012. "Empirically Supported Treatments, Evidence-Based Treatments, and Evidence-Based Practice." *Clinical Psychology*, September 8.

Durstewitz, Daniel, Georgia Koppe and Andreas Lindenberg. "Deep Neural Networks in Psychiatry." *Molecular Psychiatry* 24: 1583–98.

Egnew, Thomas. 2009. "Suffering, Meaning, and Healing: Challenges of Contemporary Medicine." *Annuals of Family Medicine* 78, no. 2 (March): 170–5.

Ekman, Paul. 2007. *Emotions Revealed, Second Edition: Recognizing Faces and Feelings to Improve Communication and Emotional Life.* New York, NY: Holt Paperbacks.

Ekstrom, S. R. 1988. "Jung's Typology and DSM-III Personality Disorders: A Comparison of Two Systems of Classification." *Journal of Analytic Psychology* 33: 329–44.

Elberty, Michael. 2019. "Knowledge Is What We Retain. Wisdom is What We Obtain," Unpublished Manuscript on Mindfulness, 12–23.

Elkins, Thomas. 2007. "The Medical Modeling Psychotherapy: Its Limitations and Failures." *Journal of Humanistic Psychology* 24 (October): 66–84.

Engel, George. 1997. "From Biomedical to Biopsychosocial: Being Scientific in the Human Domain." *Psychodynamic Psychiatry* 40, no. 3: 377–96.

Farre, Albert and Tim Rapley. 2017. "The New Old (and Old New) Medical Model: Four Decades Navigating the Biomedical and Psychosocial Understandings of Health and Illness." *Healthcare* 5, no. 4: 88. doi:10.3390/healthcare5040088

Fink, Dee. 2000. "Higher Level Learning: A Taxonomy for Identifying Different Kinds of Significant Learning." *Essays on Teaching Excellence* 11, no. 8: 13–25.

Fischer, Constance. 1994. *Individualizing Psychological Assessment: A Collaborative and Therapeutic Approach.* New York, NY: Routledge.

Fleury, Marie-Josee, Armelle Imboua, Denise Aube', Lambert Farand and Yves Lambert. 2012. "General Practitioners' Management of Mental Disorders: A Rewarding Practice with Considerable Obstacles." *BMC Family Practice* 13, no. 19: 87.

Forte, Tiago. 2017. "Moods Are the Brain's Way of Creating Momentum." *Thrive Global,* June 18, 2017. b2713bae6c2c

Frankl, Viktor. 2014. *The Will to Meaning: Foundations and Applications of Logo Therapy.* London: Penguin Group.

———. 2014. *Man's Search for Meaning.* Boston, MA: Beacon Press.

———. 2010. *The Doctor and the Soul: From Psychotherapy to Logo Therapy.* New York, NY: Vintage Books.

———. 2009. *The Unheard Cry for Meaning: Psychotherapy and Humanism.* New York, NY: Touchstone Publishers.

———. 1973. *Psychotherapy and Existentialism: Selected Papers on Logo-Therapy.* New York, NY: Pelican Books.

Freire, Jose', Marcelo Costa, Carinne Magnago, and Aldaisa Forster. 2018. "Attitudes Towards Inter- Professional Collaboration of Primary Care Teams Participating in the 'More Doctors' Program." *The Revista Latino-Americana de Enfermagem* 26 (August): 3018.

Freud, Sigmund and James Strachy.1989. *Five Lectures on Psychoanalysis.* New York, NY: W.W. Norton Company

Fritscher, Lisa. 2019. "Medical Model Use in Psychology." *Very Well Mind,* October 18, 2019.

Fuchs, Thomas and George Messas. 2019. "More Than Just Description: Phenomenology and Psychotherapy." *Psychopathology* 52: 63–6. https://doi.org/10.1159/000502266

Ghanemi, Abdelaziz. 2014. "Psychiatric Neural Networks and Neuropharmacology: Selected Advances and Novel Implications." *Saudi Pharmacological Journal* 22, no. 2 (April): 95–100.

Gladwell, Malcolm. 2007. *Blink: The Power of Thinking Without Thinking*. New York, NY: Back Bay Books.

Goleman, Daniel. 2005. *Emotional Intelligence*. New York, NY: Bantam Books.

Hafner, Hienz. 1985. "Are Mental Disorders Increasing Over Time?" *Psychopathology* 18, no. 3: 66–81.

Hansen, James. 2017. "Psychological Suffering as Message or Malady: Ideological and Cultural Contributions of Humanism." *Journal of Humanistic Psychology*, April 10. https://doi.org/10.1002/johc.12041

———. 2016. *Meaning Systems and Mental Health Culture: Critical Perspectives on Contemporary Counseling and Psychotherapy*. Lanham, MD: Lexington Books.

Hayes, Stephen. 2005. *Get Out of Your Mind & Into Your Life: The New Acceptance and Commitment Therapy*. Oakland, CA: New Harbinger.

Heidegger, Martin. 2019. *Being and Time*. Eastford, CT: Martino Fine Books.

Ho, Jeffery, Shirley Ngai, William Wu and Wai Hou. 2018. "Association Between Daily Life Experience and Psychological Well-being in People Living with Non-Psychotic Mental Disorders." *Protocol for a Systematic Review and Meta-Analysis* 4, no. 7 (June) PMID: 29369215.

Hobson, Robert. 1985. *Forms of Feeling*. London: Taylor & Francis Ltd.

Hockaday, Stacey, William Purkey and Keith Davis. 2001. "Intentionality in Helping Relationships: The Influence of Three Forms of Internal Cognitions on Behavior." *Journal of Humanistic Counseling and Education Development* 1, no. 5: 219–24.

Hubbard Timothy. 2015. "The Varieties of Momentum-Like Experience." *Psychological. Bulletin* 141, no. 6 (November): 1081–119.

Hunt Carly, Jeremy Rietschel, Bradley Hatfield and Seppo Iso-Ahola. 2013. "A Psychophysiological Profile of Winners and Losers in Sport Competition." *Sport Exercise Performance Psychology* 2, no. 3: 220–31. http://dx.doi.org/10.1037/a0031957

Hunt, Carly. 2015. "Forms of Momentum Across Time: Behavioral and Psychological." *Journal Mind Behavior* 36, no. 1 (Spring): 47–82.

Husserl, Edmund. 2014. "Ideas for a Pure Phenomenology and Phenomenology Philosophy: First Look: General Introduction to Pure Phenomenology." *Hackett Publishing Company*, March 15.

Insel, Thomas and Bruce Cuthbert. 2015. "Brain Disorders: Precisely." *Science* 348, no. 6234: 499–500. doi:10.1126/science. Aab 2358

Kays, Jill, Robin Hurley, and Katherine Taber. 2012. "The Dynamic Brain: Neuroplasticity and Mental Health." *Journal of Neuropsychiatry* 24 (April 1): 2.

Kelly, Melisa. 2018. "Putting the Parts Together to Create New Meaning." *Good Therapy*, September 19. https://www.goodtherapy.org/

Kezelman, Cathy and Pam Stavropoulos. 2012. "Practice Guidelines for Treatment of Complex Trauma and Trauma Informed Care and Service Delivery." *The Rural Monitor,* February 10, 2012.

Iacobini, Marco. 2009. *Mirroring People: The Science of Empathy and How We Connect with Others*. New York, NY: Picador Publishing.

Jacob, Karl and Vin Patel. 2014. "Classification of Mental Disorders: A Global Mental Health Perspective." *Indian Journal of Psychological Medicine* 383 (April): 1433–5. doi:10.1016/S0140-6736(13)62382-X

Jacobson, Sheri. 2016. "What is the Therapeutic Alliance and Why is it Important?" *Counseling Theory & Training*, 23 June: Harley Therapy Counseling blog.

Jensen, Dallas R. 2006. *Medical Model Influence in Counseling and Psychotherapy: Counseling Psychology Training Directors' Views.* All Theses and Dissertations, 435.

Johnson, Marcus. 2018. "4 Business Collaboration Trends That Are Changing the Way We Do Business," *Instipage Publishing*, September.

Kononov, Jake. 2012. "Identifying Locations with Potential for Accident Reductions: Use of Direct Diagnostics and Pattern Recognition Methodologies." *Sage Publications*, January 1. https://doi.org/10.3141/1784-19

Kounios, John and Mark Beeman. 2016. "The Cognitive Neuroscience of Insight." *Current Directions in Psychological Science* 18, no. 4 (August): 14.

Kumagai, Hiroshi and Akira Suda. 2010. "Identification and Functions of Pattern-Recognition Receptors." *WPI Immunology Frontier Research Center.*

Kurzwell, Raymond. 2012. *How to Create a Mind- The Secret of Human Thought Revealed.* New York: Penguin Books.

Kusnanto, Hari, Dwi Agustian and Dany Hilmanto. 2018. "Biopsychosocial Model of Illnesses in Primary Care: A Hermeneutic Literature Review." *Journal Family Med Prim Care* 20, no. 3 (May–June): 500. doi:10.4103/jfmpc.jfmpc_145_17

Lacey, Kay. 2006. "Introduction to Psychosynthesis and Its Application in Psychotherapy." *American Counseling Association*. Washington, DC.

Ladd, Peter. 2019. "The Talk Therapy Presentation." *St. Lawrence University. YouTube*, November 30.

———. 2018. *The Talk Therapy Revolution: Neuroscience, Phenomenology and Mental Health*. Lanham, MD: Lexington Books.

———. 2016. "A Scar is Not a Wound: A Metaphor for Counseling." *Counseling Today,* November 10, 2016.

———. 2013. "Knowledge vs. Wisdom in DSM Diagnosis: A Person-Centered Approach." In Gary R. Walz (ed.), *Vistas Counselor Professional and Career Development* (pp. 1–10). Washington, DC: American Counseling Association.

———. 2012. "Where is Mental Health Diagnosis Heading, And Where Does the DSM Fall Short?" *Institute of Mental Health* 29 (June).

———. 2009. *Emotional Addictions*. Lanham, MD: University Press of America.

———. 1976. *Resentment of Authority: A Phenomenological Approach.* San Diego, CA: US International University Press.

Ladd, Peter and Kyle Blanchfield. 2016. *Mediation, Conciliation and Emotions: The Role of Emotional Climate in Understanding Violence and Mental Health.* Revised Edition. Lanham, MD: Lexington Books.

Ladd, Peter and AnnMarie Churchill. 2012. *Person-Centered Diagnosis and Treatment in Mental Health: A Model for Empowering Clients.* London: Jessica Kingsley Publishers.

Lake, James. 2017. "Urgent Need for Improved Mental Health Care and a More Collaborative Model of Care." *Permanent Journal* 21 (August): 17–24. doi:7812/TPP/17-024

Larsen, Dan., William Edey and Lee Lemay. 2007. "Understanding the Role of Hope in Counseling: Exploring the Intentional Uses of Hope." *Counseling Psychology Quarterly* 20, no. 4 (December): 401–16.

Litrell, Jill. 2015. *Neuroscience for Psychologists and Other Mental Health Professionals.* New York, NY: Springer Publications.

London, Scott. 2018. *The Power of Dialogue.* http://www.scottlondon.com/articles/ondialogue.html

Mabaquiao, Napoleon. "Husserl's Theory of Intentionality." *An International Journal of Philosophy* 34, no. 1: 24–9.

MacDonald, Chloe and Kristof Mikes-Lui. 2012. *Is There a Place for Biopsychosocial Formulation in a Systemic Practice?* Cambridge: Cambridge University Press.

May, Rollo. 2003. *The Courage to Create.* New York, NY: W.W. Norton.

———.1965. "Intentionality, the Heart of Human Will." *Journal of Humanistic Psychology*. https://doi.org/10.1177/002216786500500209

McCloud, Saul. 2014. *Simply Psychology.* Manchester: University of Manchester Press.

Meeks, Thomas and Filip Jeste. 2009. "Neurobiology of Wisdom?: A Literature Review." *General Psychiatry* 66, no. 4: 355–65.

Merleau-Ponty, Maurice. 2002. *Phenomenology of Perception.* London: Routledge Classics.

———. _1992. *Sense and Non-Sense: Studies in Phenomenology and Existential Philosophy.* Chicago, IL: Northwestern University Press.

Miemis, Venessa. 2010. "Essential Skills for 21 Century Survival: Part I: Pattern Recognition." Retrieved from Emergent by Design." *Journal A Clinical Immunology* 125, no. 5 (May–June): 985–92.

Miller, William and Steven Rollnick. 2012. *Motivational Interviewing: Helping People Change.* New York, NY: Guilford Publications.

Mnookin, Robert. 1998. "Barriers to Conflict Resolution." *Alternative Dispute Resolution* 223.

Moylana, Patrick, James Lombardi and Stephen Moylanc. 2016. "Einstein's 1905 Paper on E=mc2" 131, no. 1 (January): 5–11.

Nanda Kyoto. 2009. "Mindfulness; A Lived Experienced Existential-Phenomenology Themes." *Existential Analysis* 1, no. 20 (January): 109–119.

Narkman, Robert. 2018. "See the World Through Patterns." *Psychology Today*, January 18.

Nemoroff, Charles, Daniel Weinberger, Michael Rutter, Harriet L. MacMillan, Simon Wessely, Dan J. Stein, Carmine M. Pariante, Florian Seemüller, Michael Berk, and

Gin S. Malhi. 2013. "DSM-5: A Collection of Psychiatrist Views on the Changes, Controversies, and Future Directions." *BMC Medicine* 2, no. 11: 202.

Nesse, Randolph and Dan Stein. 2012. "Towards a Genuinely Medical Model for Psychiatric Nosology." *BMC Medicine*, January 13.

Neubauer, Brian, Catherine Wittkof and Lara Varpio. 2019. "How Phenomenology Can Help Us Learn from the Experiences of Others." *Perspective in Medical Education* 8, no. 2 (April): 90–7.

Novak, Sova. 2015. "Diagnosis of Mental Illness Today and Tomorrow: A Literary Review of the Current Methods, Drawbacks, and Sociological Components of Mental Health with Regard to the Diagnosis of Mental Illness." *Portland State University.*

Pai, Anushka, Alina Suris and Carol North. 2018. "Posttraumatic Stress Disorder in the DSM 5: Controversy, Change, and Conceptual Consideration." *Medicine* 97, no. 4 (January) PMCID: PMC579439.

Parnas, Joseph and Dan Zahavi. 2002. "The Role of Phenomenology in Psychiatric Diagnosis and Classification." In Tania Gergel (ed.), *Psych Info in Psychiatric Diagnosis and Classification* (pp. 137–62). Hoboken, NJ: John Wiley & Sons Inc.

Perry, Charmain. 2016. "Medical Model vs Wellness Model." *American Counseling Association*, May.

Peterson, Tanya. 2017. "How is Schizophrenia Diagnosed? DSM-5 Diagnosis Criteria." *Healthy Place for Mental Health*, March 7, 2017.

Piaget, Jean and Brian Endler. 1972. *The Psychology of the Child.* New York, NY: Basic Books.

Polanyi, Michael. 1974. *Personal Knowledge: Toward a Post-Critical Philosophy.* Chicago, IL: University of Chicago Press.

Puder, David. 2019. "How Empathy Works And How To Improve It." *Psychology and Psychiatry Podcast*, January.

Richardson, Ronald and Donald Trepel. 2015. "Screening for Psychological and Mental Health Difficulties in Young People Who Offend: A Systematic Review and Decision Model." *Health Technology Assessment* 19, no. 1 (January).

Riddle, John. 2012. "Eye Movement Desensitization and Reprocessing is a Psychotherapy Technique Used to Treat Anxiety, PTSD, and More." *PSYCOM.*

Rogers, Carl. 2003. *Client-Centered Therapy: Its Current Practice, Implications, and Theory.* New York, NY: Robinson Publishing.

———. 1980. *A Way of Being.* New York, NY: Houghton and Mifflin.

Rogers, Carl and John Wood. 1974. *Client-Centered Theory.* Oxford: Brunner/Mazel.

Safran, Jermey, Christopher Muran and Catherine Eubanks-Carter. 2014. "Investigating the Impact of Alliance Focused Training on Interpersonal Process and Therapists' Capacity for Experiential Reflection." *Psychotherapy Research* 24: 269–85.

Samples, Bob. 2017. "Metaphoric Mind: A Celebration of Creative Consciousness." *Daily Sabah* 18, no. 6: 23–48.

Sandell, Rolf, Anna Lazar, Johan Grant, Jan Carlson, Johan Schubert and Jeanette Broberg. 2007. "Therapist Attitudes Influence Change During Treatment." *Psychotherapy Research* 17, no. 2: 196–204.

Schmidt, John. 1994. "Counselor Intentionality and Effective Helping." *Counseling and Human Services* 04-00.
Schwartz, Mel. 2017. "Integrating Your Intellect and Intuition to Achieve Wisdom." *Psychology Today*, December.
Scott, C. E. 2002. "Medard Boss." In: A. T. Tymieniecka AT. (ed.), *Phenomenology World-Wide.* (The Yearbook of Phenomenological Research), vol. 80. Dordrecht: Springer.
Selye, Hans. 1976. *The Stress of Life.* Revised edition. New York: McGraw-Hill.
Sexena, Shekha. 2019. "4 Ways to Keep the Momentum Rolling on Mental Health." *Global Competitiveness Report*, May 27.
Siegel, Daniel. 2016. *Mind: A Journey to the Heart of Being Human.* New York, NY: W.W. Norton and Company.
———. 2010. *The Mindful Brain: The Neurobiology of Well-Being.* New York, NY: W.W. Norton and Company.
Singleton, Oscar. 2014. "Change in Brainstem Gray Matter Concentration Following a Mindfulness-Based Intervention is Correlated with Improvement in Psychological Well- Being." *Frontiers Human Neuroscience* 8, no. 33 (July): 47–67.
Smith, Robert. 2012. "An Evidence-Based Patient-Centered Method Makes the Biopsychosocial Model Scientific." *American Journal of Psychiatry* 137: 535–44.
Stanislas, Dehaene. 2014 *Consciousness and the Brain.* New York, NY: Penguin Group.
Stosny, Steven. 2014. "How We Make the Same Mistakes Over and Over Again: Outgrow the Habit of Turning Setbacks into Loss and Pain into Suffering." *Psychology Today*, December.
Tartakovsky, Margarita. 2018. "The Reasons We Ruminate and How to Reduce the Cycle." *Psych Central*, July 18.
Taylor, Michael and Jon Fuchs. 1971. "Phenomenology an Alternative Approach to Diagnosis of Mental Disease." *Comprehensive Psychiatry* 12, no. 5 (September): 5–22.
Tiberius, Valerie. 2008. "Wisdom and Flexibility." In *The Reflective Life*, April. doi:10.1093/acprof:oso/9780199202867.003.0003
Tyson, Neil de Grasse. 2015. "Cosmos: A Spacetime Odyssey-Transcripts (Episode 3), When Knowledge Conquered Fear." *Cosmos*, January.
Underwood, Emily. 2019. "Brain Scans Could Help Personalize Treatment for People Who are Depressed or Suicidal." *Science*, August 20.
Valtanen, Kari. 2019. "The Psychiatrist's Role in Implementing an Open Dialogue Model of Care." *Australian Association of Family Therapy*, August 22.
Van der Kolk, Bessel. 2015. *The Body Keeps the Score: Brain, Mind, and Body in the Healing of Trauma.* New York, NY: Penguin Books.
Voros, Sebastian. 2016. "Sitting with the Demons-Mindfulness, Suffering and Existential Transformations." *Research G ate*, August. doi:10.4312/as.2016.4.2.59-83
Wade, Derick and Peter Halligan. 2017. "The Bio/Psycho/Social Model of Illness: A Model Whose Time has Come." *Rehabilitation Journal,* Sage Publications, July 21.

Walsh, Diana. 2005. “Trustworthy Leadership: Can We Be the Leaders We Need Our Students to Become?” *Institute of College Student Values*, February 5.

Wamphold, Bruce. 2000. *The Great Psychotherapy Debate*. New York, NY: Routledge.

Wasserman, Theodore and Lori Wasserman. 2019. “Understanding Functional Neural Networks.” Part of *Neural Network Model: Applications and Implications*. New York, NY: Springer Publishing.

Waters, Brad. 2015. “23 Mental Health Professionals Interviewed About Their Jobs.” *Psychology Today*, June 24.

Websters Dictionary. 2019. “Nuances.” *Merriam-Webster Inc.*

White, Tracie. 2016. “How Neuroscience Could Determine Your Mental Health Treatment.” *Precision Health*, February.

Williams, Mark and Danny Penhman. 2012. *Mindfulness: An Eight-Week Plan for Finding Peace in a Frantic World*. Emmaus, PA: Rodale Books.

Willis, Olivia. 2018. “Psychiatrists, Psychologists and Counsellors: Who to See for your Mental Health Issues.” *ABC Health & Wellbeing*, October.

Wittchen, Hans-Ulrich. 2003. “Mental Disorders in Primary Care.” *Clinical Neuroscience* 5, no. 2 (June): 115. PMC3181625.

Wooley, Anita. 2015. “Collective Intelligence and Group Performance.” *Current Directions in Psychological Science* 24, no. 6:420–4.

Zhu, Ex. 2018. “Exposure-Based Therapy Changes Amygdala and Hippocampus Resting-State Functional Connectivity in Patients with Posttraumatic Stress Disorder.” *National Institute of Health* 35, no. 10 (October): 974–84. doi: 10.1002/da.22816.

Index

About the Author

Peter D. Ladd, PhD, LMHC, has been a tenured faculty member at St. Lawrence University in the Graduate School of Education for over thirty-five years. He coordinated the Mental Health Counseling Program—an existential phenomenological approach to mental health counseling. Also, he has worked for thirty-eight years with St. Lawrence University's satellite graduate school program on the Akwesasne Mohawk Reservation. Over his career, he resided as a graduate assistant for Viktor Frankl in the mid-1970s. He worked with Carl Rogers as a contributing author for the book, *Freedom to Learn for the Eighties*, and attended Duquesne University where he studied existential phenomenology. He is an award-winning author and this will be his fourteenth book, all with a phenomenological emphasis, and one winning a national book award. A related book to this current is *The Talk Therapy Revolution: Neuroscience, Phenomenology and Mental Health* by Lexington Books (2018). He has written numerous articles in the areas of addictions counseling, mental health counseling, relationship counseling, and conflict resolution. Dr. Ladd also works on the Akwesasne Mohawk Reservation where he established two mental health counseling centers and was the licensed clinical supervisor for the Tekanikonrahwa:kon Holistic Health and Wellness Program, working closely with Native Healers from the Tribe. He is presently working as a trauma consultant for the St. Regis Mohawk Tribe and has formed a trauma-informed care center dealing with domestic violence, sex trafficking, and PTSD and other traumas.

www.ingramcontent.com/pod-product-compliance
Ingram Content Group UK Ltd.
Pitfield, Milton Keynes, MK11 3LW, UK
UKHW041843031026
15587UKWH00002B/968

9 781793 619013